Essential Texts in Chinese Medicine

by the same author

The Great Intent
Acupuncture Odes, Songs and Rhymes
Richard Bertschinger
ISBN 978 1 84819 132 7
eISBN 978 0 85701 111 4

Everyday Qigong Practice
Richard Bertschinger
ISBN 978 1 84819 117 4
eISBN 978 0 85701 097 1

Yijing, Shamanic Oracle of China
A New Book of Change
Translated by Richard Bertschinger
ISBN 978 1 84819 083 2
eISBN 978 0 85701 066 7

The Secret of Everlasting Life
The First Translation of the Ancient Chinese Text on Immortality
Richard Bertschinger
ISBN 978 1 84819 048 1
eISBN 978 0 85701 054 4

RICHARD BERTSCHINGER

ESSENTIAL TEXTS
in Chinese Medicine

The Single Idea in the Mind of the Yellow Emperor

FOREWORD BY ALLEN PARROTT

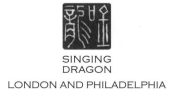

SINGING
DRAGON
LONDON AND PHILADELPHIA

First published in 2015
by Singing Dragon
an imprint of Jessica Kingsley Publishers
73 Collier Street
London N1 9BE, UK
and
400 Market Street, Suite 400
Philadelphia, PA 19106, USA

www. singingdragon. com

Library of Congress Cataloging in Publication Data
Bertschinger, Richard, author.
  Essential texts in Chinese medicine : the single idea in
the mind of the Yellow Emperor / Richard
Bertschinger.
      p. ; cm.
  Translation of and commentary on the Nei jing zhi yao of
Ming doctor and scholar Li Zhongzi, alongside
the original Chinese, with a number of additional texts from the Huang di nei jing.
  Includes bibliographical references.
  ISBN 978-1-84819-162-4 (alk. paper)
  I. Li, Zhongzi, 1588-1655. Nei jing zhi yao. II. Li, Zhongzi,
1588-1655. Nei jing zhi yao. English III. Huangdi
nei jing. Selections. IV. Huangdi nei jing. English Selections. V. Title.
  [DNLM: 1. Huangdi nei jing. 2. Medicine, Chinese
Traditional--history. 3. Medicine, Chinese
Traditional--methods. 4. Manuscripts, Medical--history. WZ 294]
  R127. 1
  610. 951--dc23
                                2014021760

British Library Cataloguing in Publication Data
A CIP catalogue record for this book is available from the British Library

ISBN 978 1 84819 162 4
eISBN 978 0 85701 135 0

Printed and bound by Bell & Bain Ltd, Glasgow

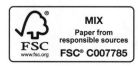

At the stillpoint of the turning world…

Gia-fu Feng

The Tao gave birth to One,
One gives birth to two,
Two gives birth to three,
Three gives birth to the ten thousand things.
The ten thousand things all bear Yin on their backs
And embrace the Yang,
Infused with a single breath they form an easy harmony.

Laozi, Chapter 42

CONTENTS

Foreword by Allen Parrott.   11

A NOTE ON THE TEXT   13

Introduction.   15
    1. The History of the Yellow Emperor's Medical Classic. *16*
    2. Philosophical Roots in the Neijing *17*
    3. Yinyang and Wuxing. *23*
    4. Li Zhongzi, His Compilation and the Quietly Enquiring Mind   *31*
    5. A World Refracted through Chinese Language. *38*
    6. Claude Levi-Strauss and the Untamed Mind *42*
    7. A Logic of Tangible Qualities. *45*
    8. Conclusion: A Divide in Medical Thinking. *49*
    Characters in the Introduction *51*

I   The Arts and Ways of a Good Life   52
    Key Ideas. *52*
    1. The Yellow Emperor Questions his Counsellor. *54*
    2. A Message from the Ancients *56*
    3. They Represented the Arts and Ways of Life *58*
    4. The Rhythm of the Seasons *62*
    5. The Energy of the Yang Stored up. *67*
    6. The Practice of Advancing the Yang. *70*
    7. Taoist Yoga *73*
    8. The Sages Treated those Well, not those Sick *75*
    9. The Character of the Malign Xie or Thief-Wind. *76*
    Questions for Review of Chapter I. *78*
    Characters in Chapter I. *79*

II   Yin and Yang   80
    Key Ideas. *80*
    1. Yin and Yang, the Way of the Skies and Earth. *81*
    2. Yin and Yang, Water, Fire, Qi and Flavours *85*
    3. Left and Right as different as North and South *92*
    4. Yin and Yang in the Skies and Man *94*
    5. The Crucial Importance of the Yang Needing Rest. *97*
    Questions for Review of Chapter II *99*
    Characters in Chapter II *100*

III   Examining the Colour 101

Key Ideas. *101*

1. Purity, Brightness, Colour and Complexion *102*

2. The Bright-lit Hall, the Physiognomy of Face *105*

3. The Basis of Health in the Face. *114*

Questions for Review of Chapter III. *117*

Characters in Chapter III. *117*

IV   The Quiet Pulse 118

Key Ideas. *118*

1. The Method of the Pulse Exam *120*

2. If a Single Pulse Stands Out *124*

3. The Primacy of the Pulse. *125*

4. In Attending to the Pulse. *126*

5. In Spring, the Pulse is in the Liver *128*

6. The Healthy, Sick and Fatal Pulses *133*

7. The Arrival of the Fatal Pulse *138*

8. The Ultimate Tool. *143*

9. A Common Fault in the Pulse Exam *145*

Questions for Review of Chapter IV. *146*

Characters in Chapter IV. *147*

V   The *Zangfu* and *Wuxing* 148

Key Ideas. *148*

1. The Offices of the Zangfu. *150*

2. The Zang and their Associations *153*

3. Directions and Elemental Associations *156*

4. Further Elemental Forms and Wuxing Science *159*

5. The Faculties of the Self, and their Injuries *167*

6. Physical Functions in Life and Death. *170*

Questions for Review of Chapter V *173*

Characters in Chapter V *174*

VI   Channels and Collaterals 175

Key Ideas. *175*

1. The Form and Length of the Channels *176*

Question for Review of Chapter VI *189*

Characters in Chapter VI. *189*

VII   Patterns of Treatment. 190

Key Ideas. *190*

1. Yin and Yang, the Rule and Pattern *192*

2. The Seed in Sickness *194*

3. *Mind, Body and Disease* 196
4. *Regional Types, Regional Medicines.* 198
5. *Treatment with Herbals, Foodstuffs and Flavours* 202
6. *How Foodstuffs and Medicines can do Harm* 208
7. *Therapeutic Actions, How to Treat* 209
8. *Five Faults Made during Treatment* 212
9. *The Ultimate Task* 215
Questions for Review of Chapter VII 217
Characters in Chapter VII 217

VIII   The Method of Needling 219
Key Ideas. 219
1. *Origins of Five Element Acupuncture.* 221
2. *Opening Chapter of the Lingshu* 226
3. *The Method* 231
4. *Acupuncture: Treatment by Sun, Moon and Planets.* 233
5. *He Who Observes the Minutest of Changes* 236
6. *Acupuncture: Technique, Reducing and Reinforcing.* 238
7. *Acupuncture: What is Meant by the Spirit* 241
8. *Four Common Failings in Treatment* 243
Questions for Review of Chapter VIII 245
Characters in Chapter VIII 245

IX   Pathology. 246
Key Ideas. 246
1. *A Typology of Conditions.* 248
2. *Elemental, Seasonal and Dietary Injuries.* 251
3. *Elemental Forms and Body Isomorphism* 254
4. *A Complete Explanation of the Full or Weak* 259
5. *Cold and Heat, Yin and Yang, Inner and Outer* 262
6. *The Five Full, the Five Weak.* 265
7. *On the Temperament.* 267
8. *How Heat Represents in the Face.* 270
9. *On the Progression of Fevers* 272
10. *On Various Kinds of Pain.* 275
11. *On Bi Immobility Syndromes* 279
12. *On Dreaming 1* 282
13. *On Dreaming 2* 284
14. *Times of Dying: Channel Collapse* 288
15. *Times of Dying: Seasonal Collapse.* 292
16. *The Collapse of the Channels* 294
Questions for Review of Chapter IX 296
Characters in Chapter IX. 297

APPENDIX A: CLINICAL COSMOLOGY   298
APPENDIX B: XUE SHENGBAI'S DISCOVERY OF
LI ZHONGZI'S WORK.   303
SELECT BIBLIOGRAPHY AND SOURCES.   307
NOTES   309

List of Tables

Fundamental Chinese Virtues in Medicine   21
Correspondences with Nature.   25
Human Body Correspondences   26
Elemental *Yijing* Trigrams   27
Eulogy on Humankind   61
Rhythm of Life   66
The *Yinyang*   84
A Vigorous Fire, a Lesser Fire   91
Yinyang in the Heavens   95
Yinyang in the Human Body   96
Flowering of the Qi   104
Physiognomy of Face   113
Fatality in the Face and Eyes.   116
The Pulse   127
The Seasonal Pulse.   132
Ministries of the *Zangfu*   152
Traditional Correspondences of the *Zangfu*   155
Pentatonic Tone, Element and Aspect   165
Five Directions with Traditional Associations   166
The Yin and Yang   193
Propriety of the Cure   197
Treatments Tailored to Locality and Background   201
Herbal Actions Must Accord   206
Acting in Accord with the Condition   207
The Resonance of Sky and Earth   235
A Simple Pathology   250
Five Elemental Forms of People   258
Qi Strata.   269
Weakness Results in Dreaming   283
Fullness Results in Dreaming   287
The Reversing Qi Results in Dreaming   287

Foreword

Richard Bertschinger's work on these important Chinese texts deserves to become an 'essential text' for medicine in the 21st century. His book has achieved a rare three-way combination: scholarly for academics, accessible for students, and relevant to practitioners. The entire acupuncture community will be grateful for his labours.

But I also believe his mention of Mencius and Confucian thought has lessons for a very different readership. It is more than two millennia since Hippocrates urged doctors to consider the person as a whole, but this wisdom seems to have been lost in modern medicine – or at least temporarily mislaid. Parts of this book should be required reading for the entire body of Western practitioners, because it re-states key human values and consequent approaches to medical practice that are genuinely 'complementary' and beneficial to scientific biomedicine.

Through personal experience, I have long believed that traditional acupuncture has much that can actually enhance and improve Western medical practice. Richard Bertschinger's book illustrates conclusively that it has much more to offer than treatment for pain and muscular-skeletal conditions. It articulates some of the ancient wisdom on medical ethics, patient care and practitioner development – 'rightness in action' Mencius called it – still needed by healthcare professionals in the 21st century, and which could usefully be the basis of much continuing professional development.

The book also provides practitioners with a very useful set of deep metaphors, taken from nature, society, and life as it is lived. It does not start with the human body as a kind of machine or complex set of mechanisms, chemical elements or physical forces only properly 'known' in the ivory tower of the scientific laboratory. It offers a better approach, therefore, to the messy, real life of medicine where mind and body are inseparable and when the machine metaphor breaks down and fails to deliver. 'Rightness in action', indeed.

Now that China is set to overtake the USA as the world's largest economic power, is it so strange to take a lesson from their traditions? Richard Bertschinger's book would be a good place for Western doctors to start this serious learning process.

Allen Parrott
Formerly, Lead Accreditation Officer,
British Acupuncture Accreditation Board

A NOTE ON THE TEXT

A differing world-view, a different sensibility in medicine; that is what is presented in these texts. Yet when I first read Li Zhongzi's *Cornerstone to the Neijing* (1642) in the summer of 1986, I felt no difference between us, no difficulty in understanding what he was saying. It was as if I had found a friend at my elbow, a trusted guide and mentor by my side. For publication I have abridged his work slightly, notably in the pathology section (Chapter IX), to keep it relevant and accessible to modern practitioners. I have also added a little to the choice of texts; some on acupuncture, on the spirit in needling and diagnosis, on place, and on Five Element typology. I have also leaned heavily on modern Chinese editions of the *Huangdi Neijing*, as well on the Japanese commentaries of the Tamba family (see Select Bibliography and Sources), and the exacting inspiration of Gia-fu Feng (1919–1985). The enticing animal designs that accompany each translation come from a silk-embroidered altar-cloth found in a Warring States (c. 300 BCE) tomb from Hubei Province, contemporary with the *Huangdi Neijing*. I have also gained support from many, to whom my grateful thanks: Derek Woodward, Professor Man Fong Mei (Benny Mai), Alan Hext, Sara Hicks, Professor Elisabeth Hsu, Dr Tim Gordon, Dr Allen Parrott, Dr Jidong Wu, Russell Chapman, Jane Robinson, Lesley Jenkins, Dr Barry Nicholls, Trish Robinson, Paul Hougham, Dr Charlotte Paterson – none of whom, of course, should be held responsible for my faults and errors, which are entirely of my own making.

Introduction

The aim of these texts is to provide an accessible view of the fundamental writings of classical Chinese medicine and to give an indication of that peculiar fusion of medical thought and noted sensibility, which is so Chinese. I have used exclusively the *Huangdi Neijing* or *Yellow Emperor's Medical Classic* (texts mostly assembled c. 200 BCE–200 CE) – the well-spring of Chinese medicine for two thousand years. As a result of pondering these texts and ideas in my own practice, I have come to a clearer knowledge of the immediacy and joy of this wonderful medicine. People get well quicker and that is everything we want. And, in addition, I have begun to understand the simplicity and subtlety residing in Chinese thinking. But more about that later.

The method of reasoning behind the ideas expressed in the *Neijing* is not 'scientific' in the common sense of the word. Its particular feature is an organic logic, which may be called loosely 'associative' – or, more usually, 'correlative' thinking. For instance, the heart is not just seen as an intricate double-action pump (mechanical) but as the supreme 'ruler', or 'lord and master' (that is, associative, pictorial), within the body. The liver is not just the seat of the body's metabolism and detoxification but a 'military commander', or general, of the body's whole forces. Indeed, the whole body and its functions may be seen to be run as a kingdom or state. This method of reasoning, more poetic and richer in imaginative thinking, is due to the features of the Chinese language – it nominally includes 'words', but also 'idea-centres' (characters), which allow a freer range of thought. This would usually accompany the 'primitive', what we might call 'unschooled' mind – but is a thinking no less vigorous or analytic than that used in Western science, even if it never adopted Aristotelian logic – and, more emphatically, the law of the excluded middle (where a thing could be A or not A, but never possessed of the qualities of both).

1. The History of the Yellow Emperor's Medical Classic

The *Neijing* (*Yellow Emperor's Medical Classic*) is the longest surviving text on medical theory from China, surviving to the present day. It consists of two volumes: the *Suwen* (*Basic Questions*) and the *Lingshu* (*The Spiritual Crux*) – both covering medical theory and practice of the day. We know conclusively that the body of the text first appeared, in some form, around the period of the later Warring States (472–221 BCE) and Han (206 BCE–220 CE), and is part of a tradition acknowledging as patron the Yellow Emperor (a mythical appellation): its style similar to a number of works put together at the same and adjoining period. It was also quoted extensively in the earliest book ever to be devoted exclusively to acupuncture – Huang Fumi's *Zhenjiu Jiayi Jing* (*An ABC of Acupuncture and Moxibustion*), dated conclusively to 282 CE.

Yet the quest for an *authentic* text has proved fruitless. Not one of the editions now extant can be said to be the Han original. Each is a mix of smaller 'primary texts' and compilations. This is why the work so readily lends itself to adaptation.

David Keegan has demonstrated that the *Neijing* was made up of many smaller texts with different authors. He sees it as a record of separate schools and approaches. These form lineages which reveal the contexts of the medical theorizing of the time. Thus the *Neijing* cannot be understood as a single coherent work. It is a compilation – in fact a compilation of compilations. The accepted view is that the *Huangdi Neijing* was probably written over a century or more and brought together in the first century BCE, or early first century CE.

Keegan suggests, on the internal evidence of certain chapters, that they were put together by physicians in order to teach students, who received the texts during a formal ceremony of transmission under oath. This meeting with the master was conducted under a binding contract to take great care of and preserve the integrity of the teachings.

Oral transmission was central. An average student's 'work-book' was integral to the craft he was being taught – but eventually, this process produced families of texts later assembled into the *Neijing*. Furthermore, the differing versions of the *Neijing* now extant are *also* products of a process of compilation. Each editor, thereafter, rearranged and made up a portfolio of texts and readings to give authenticity to their approach – and thus create a lineage.

As to the choice of texts given below, I have based my selection on that of the Ming physician Li Zhongzi, using his *Neijing Zhiyao* digest or *A Cornerstone to the Neijing* (published in 1642). I have included about four-fifths of his material, and some of his commentary – much of which was lifted, anyway, from his teacher Zhang Jiebin. I have also added passages on the art and spirit of needling, the origins of *wuxing* ('five element') science and personality types, as I have seen fit; and also a glimpse of the prolific Chinese commentaries, essential reading for a correct understanding of the text. I have also pointed out instances where the text is doubtful, using four or five of the versions readily available (see Select Bibliography and Sources). Li's *Cornerstone* is still widely read in China. Over the last 300 years it has served as a popular introduction to medical studies, and was even influential during the revamping of Chinese medicine in post-revolutionary China (c. 1950s). Li Zhongzi, a busy physician, somehow managed to condense the voluminous texts of the original *Neijing* into a hundredth their size, whilst preserving their irreducible message.

2. Philosophical Roots in the Neijing

We cannot understand the natural medicine of the Han and Warring States without first learning about the Confucian age during which it was born. The ancient world of the Zhou dynasty, leading into the period of the Warring States, formed the background for many of the later Han dynasty's medical texts. The Zhou were decidedly aristocratic. Theirs was the age which was to provide the seedbed for the Confucian–Taoist hodge-podge which made up classical Chinese thought. The early Zhou (the dynasty is said to have been founded c. 1060 BCE) were a prosperous feudal and agricultural people, ruled by the hegemony of the Zhou tribe – which meant a strictly aristocratic line of succession. Such a genesis to the text makes the following opening lines to Chapter V understandable:

> The heart is the office of the lord and master. A clear mind is his duty. The lungs are the officials of communications. Government and regulation are their duty. The liver is the official of the military commander. Plotting and planning are his duty. The gallbladder is the official of inner integrity. Making decisions and judgements are his duty. The 'middle chest' is the office of the messengers. Joy and pleasure are his duty. The spleen and stomach are the officials of the granaries. All foodstuffs are their duty. The large intestines are the officials of conveyances. Change and transformation are their duty. The small intestines are the officials in charge of 'receiving fullness'. The transformation of materials is their duty. The kidneys are the officers in charge of creating vigour. Ingenuity and skill are their duty.

But eventually the feudal system broke down under the impact of many irrepressible forces – the 'warring states'. These states, being feudal aristocracies, were losing their power, while the peasants, who had been serfs to their overlords, were gaining freedom and independence. Many states were swallowed up by a few, more powerful. As the social fabric was torn asunder, the military was diffused, hereditary titles fell, and the knowledge which had previously been the province of the aristocracy became available to all.

This period, stretching from the birth of Confucius (551 BCE) until the time of the ruthless Legalist Han Feizi (died 233 BCE), was an extremely fertile time for Chinese thought. Three centuries of turmoil furthered philosophical development, and certainly provided a fertile soil in which the ideas of *yinyang* and *wuxing* could grow. Yet many looked back longingly to the stability of the early Zhou. They had a fond regard for older codes of behaviour: the rules of propriety regulating social relations between ruler and minister, father and son, and so on; that is, due reverence to ancestors, and the possession of a natural and easy sense of right and wrong. These were the ideas that morphed into Confucian thinking. Add a respect for the 'old wisdom' – the oral tradition – and you have the basic ingredients for the rough-hewn virtues of early Confucianism. Such a regard for 'the ancients' 古 *gu* can be seen in the first chapter of the *Neijing* – with its harking back to a period of High Romance.

> The people of old, they understood the Way – they modelled themselves on the Yin and Yang and were at peace with the arts of destiny. Their eating and drinking were in moderation. They rose and retired at a regular hour. They neither had wild ideas, nor wearied themselves at work. Thus they were able to keep body and soul together and so attain the end of their natural span, one hundred years, and then pass away. The people of this age are not the same.

In 551 BCE, when Confucius was born, the Zhou were but a memory and the government had degenerated into petty squabbling and conflict. A final solution was not found until the supreme victory and short rule of the Qin (221–207 BCE); which established a 'reign of terror', albeit brief, founded upon the philosophy of Han Feizi, who had died somewhat earlier.

It was the Qin who standardised the Chinese script, weights and measures, and the widths of carriage axles (to stop heavy wheels rutting the roads). But, more notoriously, they also 'burnt the books', save only those on medicine, divination and agriculture, and buried alive any number of dissenting scholars, as well as rebuilding the Great Wall. All was symptomatic of a cultural watershed – and from this time on, there was to be a gradual consolidation. It is not too much to say that all Chinese thought was built upon the philosophical foundations laid by the schools of the Warring States.

Confucius – the best known philosopher of the Eastern world – regarded himself as a restorer of the old. He called himself a narrator, not a creator of regulatory mores and customs. Yet in the next few centuries, others went further. For example, Mencius (c. 300 BCE) saw the need for, and developed, virtues of *jen* 仁, 'love, kindness', *yi* 義, 'rightness in action', *li* 禮, 'a sense of propriety' and *zhi* 智, 'wisdom'. All have a relevance to the thought and morality embedded in the *Neijing*.

It was Mencius who, most importantly, made an appeal to the innate goodness of the 'heart' 心 *xin* (or 'mind'). In a famous passage he says:

> All men have a mind which cannot bear to see the suffering of others…even today, if someone suddenly sees a child about to fall into a well, they will without exception experience a feeling of alarm or distress. This will not be as a way to gain the favour of the child's parents, nor to seek the praise of the neighbours and friends, nor that they feel so because they dislike a reputation that they are unvirtuous.

He means that the good heart is our natural birthright. As Confucius had said formerly, 'reciprocity' is the watchword. Mencius thus established the Confucian principles of *jen*, kindness, *yi,* rightness, *li*, propriety and *zhi*, wisdom, finding them in our own personal feelings of compassion, shame, humility and a sense of right and wrong. Mencius believed these qualities formed the natural bent of the heart – a heart not able to bear the sufferings of others. He goes on to say:

> From this example we can see that a feeling of compassion is essential to man, a feeling of shame is essential to man, a

feeling of humility is essential to man, and a sense of right and wrong is essential to man; the feeling of compassion is the beginning of kindness, the feeling of shame is the beginning of righteousness, the feeling of humility is the beginning of propriety, and the sense of right and wrong is the beginning of wisdom. Man has these four beginnings, just as he has his four limbs.

These four fundamental virtues formed the backbone of Chinese medical ethics.

FUNDAMENTAL CHINESE VIRTUES IN MEDICINE

a feeling of compassion, bringing kindness	a feeling of shame, bringing right action	a feeling of humility, bringing propriety	a sense of right and wrong, bringing wisdom
仁 jen	義 yi	禮 li	智 zhi

He concludes:

And when people, having these four principles, yet say of themselves that they cannot develop them, they play the thief with their very selves, and those that say of their prince that he cannot develop them, they play the thief with their prince. Since all people have these four principles in themselves, let them know how to give them all their full development and completion. Then it will be like a fire starting to burn, or a spring beginning to burst forth. Let them have their full development, and they will have sufficient time to love and protect all within the four seas. Let them be denied their development, and they will not have sufficient even to serve their own parents.

These virtues identify the natural development of our own humanity and potential. Yet they are not to be emulated in themselves, or worked at or even thought about (as will be clear later) – rather they naturally arise if we devote effort to our own behavioural and physical cultivation.

The Qin, who first unified China, were only destined to reign 20 years. The Han, who followed hard on their heels, stood in direct contrast. They ushered in both a time of expansion – as their borders spread towards Korea and central Asia – and an age of scholarship, as the literati of a new China struggled to recover and preserve the thought of the previous few centuries, which had so very nearly been lost. To the Han, the texts of the past must have seemed to be fast fading and vanishing from sight. The Han was founded in 202 BCE. Yet by the time of Emperor Wudi (140–87 BCE), their first really stable ruler, these classical revisions had created the officially recognised philosophical schools of the time.

The Han was a time for retrospective scholarship and compilations. The old literature was understood in terms of their own thinking. Indeed it is not too much to say that if it were not for the efforts of the Han editors, a knowledge of China's ancient past would have been lost, for all time. It is still through their early work that we study and translate these texts to this day. They were destined to become the classics of Chinese literature. The *Changes* (*Yijing*), the *Histories* (*Shujing*), the *Poems* (*Shijing*), the *Rites* (*Liji*) and the *Spring and Autumn Annals* (*Chunqiu*) of the later Zhou are only the best known of an extensive Han reworking of much of what has subsequently become known as the Confucian canon. Thus it was natural for the *Neijing* to be cast in the same mould. The work is staged as a drama between semi-legendary personages (the Emperor and his advisors) discussing the need for medical reform – just as had taken place in history, poetry, astronomy and so on. New medical theories and ideas were introduced and treated under the guise of the old. For instance, in its opening paragraphs, the august Emperor is questioning his minister-physician Qi Bo:

> The Yellow Emperor said: 'I have heard that the men of ancient times lived through a hundred springs and autumns, yet they remained active and did not reach senility. The men of the

present day only reach half that age and yet are sen
society and age so very different? Or have I missed s
Qi Bo replied: 'The men of ancient times, they
the Way, they modelled themselves on the *yinyang* and were
at peace with the arts of destiny. Their eating and drinking
were in moderation, they rose and retired at regular hours; they
neither had wild ideas, nor wearied themselves at their work.
Thus they were able to keep body and soul together and so
attain the end of their natural span – one hundred years – and
then pass away. The men of the present day are not the same.
They drink liquor to excess; they take wild ideas as the norm.
When drunk they perform the act of love, seeking to exhaust
their qi and waste their lives. They do not know how to be
content. They have no time to control their thinking, looking
only for what cheers, not for the joys of health. They rise and
retire at any time and thus, at only fifty, are already senile. '

Reading these early texts it is clear that the thinkers of the Warring
States, and before, were strongly paternalistic, influenced by
primitive thought. Dependent for their very survival on a correct
understanding of the seasons, planting and the weather, they
saw the skies above as their 'supreme authority' 帝 *di* – echoing
the absolute rule of the Emperor. But by the time of the Han
reunification, the skies (Yang) had found a partner in the earth
(Yin). Thus there arose a more flexible, people-centred world-
view involving both Heaven and Earth; which eventually led to
the idea that there are two main 'metaphysical' agents working
in our world, the 'Yin' and the 'Yang', the arbiters of all things –
including our medical destiny.

3. Yinyang and Wuxing

At this point it would be natural to introduce the two basic
themes which permeate the *Neijing*'s scientific thinking – the
yinyang 陰陽 and *wuxing* 五行 – usually translated as Yin and Yang
and the Five Elements. A consideration of their ideas will enable

us to understand how Han physicians worked. Most scholars are sceptical about the terms *yinyang* and *wuxing* stretching back any further than around 300 BCE, although the seeds of their thought were around. Ma Boying has shown that Yin and Yang, in a concrete sense, permeated 'warring states' thinking. But the man who has most been credited with their development is the philosopher Zou Yan. There were three scholars with the surname Zou, who lived in the state of Qi and sustained and augmented these ideas during the latter period of the Warring States. They created a unified system of correspondences, feeding all kinds of observations into a *yinyang/wuxing* matrix; creating, as it were, a grand and majestic allegory of interaction between all natural and human forces. Fung Yu-lan puts forward the interesting idea that because the state of Qi bordered on the sea, their inhabitants were often hearing about new and strange events. They were apparently noted for their 'fabulous and fanciful stories'. Perhaps such a variety of stimuli led to an attempted ordering – such as that offered by the *yinyang* and *wuxing* system. Needham suggests that these states might also have been the repositories of ancient shamanism, migrating into these areas from the north and south. This giant system, so well represented in the *Suwen* (especially Chapters 4 and 5), became the cornerstone of reasoning in the Chinese sciences. Each 'element' or 'force' 行 *xing* had its period of flourishing and a period of decline – everything had its winter and its summer. Both natural and human events were explained through Yin and Yang, and when further divided into the 'Five Forces' *wuxing* – wood–growth, fire–flame, earth–soil, metal–precious and water–fluidity – their tool was applicable to all. Its genius was that it brought *relationships* to the fore – rather than *substance*. The universe was *a single system of interlocking forces*. One might say that this was the 'single idea' in the mind of the Yellow Emperor.

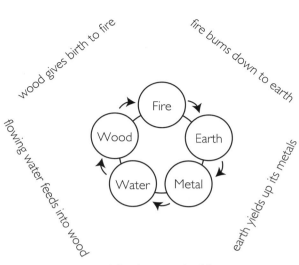

The *wuxing* (Five Element) cycle

Let me append two tables of common correspondences here, both from the *Neijing*.

CORRESPONDENCES WITH NATURE

	east	south	central	west	north
colour	blue-green	red	yellow	white	black
foodstuff	sour	bitter	sweet	pungent	salty
class	vegetation	fire	soil	metals	water
animal	cockerel	goat	ox	horse	swine
grains	wheat	millet	panicled millet	rice	peas and beans
planet	Jupiter	Mars	Saturn	Venus	Mercury
sound	*jue*	*zhi*	*gong*	*shang*	*yu*
number	8	7	5	9	6
odour	rank	scorched	fragrant	rotten	stale

HUMAN BODY CORRESPONDENCES

	liver	heart	spleen	lungs	kidneys
opens into	eye	ear	mouth	nostrils	two lower openings
sickness	fright	inner organs	root of tongue	the back	between the muscles
rests in	sinews	vessels	flesh	skin and hair	bones
body odour	rank	scorched	fragrant	rotten	stale

A correspondence between human behaviour and nature (especially the seasons) is also apparent in the early Chinese almanac, the *Yue Ling* or *Monthly Ordinances* (contained within the Confucian classic, the *Book of Rites*), compiled during the early Han:

> …each of the 'Five Powers' has its period of ascendance during the four seasons of the year. Thus the power in ascendance in spring is wood; in summer it is fire; in autumn it is metal; and in winter it is water. The places where the Emperor lives, the colours of his clothes, the kinds of food he eats, and the general conduct of his government are all rigidly determined according to the Power in ascendance during that particular month of the year.

This natural sequencing of *yinyang* is the true bedrock of Chinese natural science. But what is most surprising is that it is still used, unchanged, in contemporary texts – such as the books used in the present Chinese medical colleges teaching acupuncture and herbal medicine.

A modern acupuncture textbook from Beijing states:

> The theory of yin-yang holds that every object or phenomenon in the universe consists of two opposite aspects, namely, yin and yang, which are at once in conflict and in interdependence; further, that this relation between yin and yang is the universal law of the material world, the principle and source of the existence of myriads of things, and the root cause for the flourishing and perishing of things.

This could have been taken verbatim from the opening lines to the *Grand Discourse on the Resonant Phenomena of Yin and Yang* (*Suwen* 5):

> Yin and Yang form the Way of the skies and earth. They make up the rules and pattern for the myriad creatures; they are the father and mother of all change and transformation, the root origin of living and killing. They are the treasury of a clear mind.

The Han scholars developed the tools of *yinyang* and *wuxing* into a way of classifying all data. It was a giant bureaucracy for the pigeon-holing of experience. They were a different people to the early Zhou, the feudal aristocrats. The Han possessed a spirit of enquiry – a desire to investigate, systematise, separate out and classify, and an urge to know the whys and wherefores of the world.

Most crucial to this vision of a 'mutual interaction' 相应 *xiangying* between things were the texts of the *Yijing, Classic of Change*. These writings made use of a solid Yang line (—) to indicate firmness and union, and a weak or broken Yin line (--) to indicate dis-union or yielding, put together in pairs; then in threes (the three-line 'trigrams'; see below); and then doubled up to form sixes (six-line 'hexagrams') to form a calculus of 64 six-line figures. These figures represented the 384 possible 'changes' in the universe and became fundamental to much of Chinese science. I follow this idea up later.

ELEMENTAL *YIJING* TRIGRAMS

Heaven	Earth	Thunder	Mountain	Wind	Marsh	Fire	Water
☰	☷	☳	☶	☴	☱	☲	☵
Yang	Yin	Moving	Stillness	Entering	Passing	Light	Dark

However, this simple science of solid and broken lines (Yin and Yang) was not to everyone's liking – although it did encourage a 'sympathetic' manner in medicine, for a Chinese doctor would look for resonances and dissonances between phenomena just as he or she looked for matching lines in, or between, trigrams or hexagrams. Thus he or she could further work at his or her *wuxing* and *yinyang* acumen – leading to a greater power and understanding in diagnosis and treatment.

Health comes from a harmony or accord between Yin and Yang; while sickness means disharmony or discord. This is well illustrated in the passage quoted earlier, depicting the internal organs as 'ministers at court'. The passage concludes: '...all in all, there are twelve officials, if they cannot agree with each other, they are lost. ' In other words: seeing the body as a political entity, the body's integrity would be lost. When the ruler and ministers listen to each other, the country might be saved; while if they neglect their duty, the country (or body) will be lost. Describing the pulses, *Suwen* 20 states:

> One on its own is small, is sickness;
> One on its own is large, is sickness;
> One on its own is fast, is sickness;
> One on its own is slow, is sickness;
> One on its own is hot, is sickness;
> One on its own is cold, is sickness;
> One on its own sunken, is sickness.

A pulse standing out 'on its own' under the finger signifies something unusual or discordant – seemingly different to the touch. Note how simple this is. A practical truth; not a 'thinking process'. It is based upon a logic of the concrete. Not a one-to-one correspondence with the world – but a meshing together of finger and object, in the sense of something 'workable' in the real world, in the fist-hittable, material world. In the very first chapter of the *Neijing* ('The Natural Behaviour of Those of Ancient Times', *Suwen* 1) this is shown by eulogising about those people who use their full range of human skills and abilities – the 'truly human' or 'realised' 真人 *zhenren*, a Confucian and Taoist ideal. For instance:

...and then there were the Adepts, their lofty virtue reached its fulfilment in their methods (*dao*). They lived in peace with Yin and Yang, and were in harmony with the four seasons. They left the common world, away from all custom, building up a purity to fashion their thinking. They wandered 'twixt the skies and earth, they looked and listened at all points of the compass – finally this promoted their destiny and they became strong. This returned them to being as real people of substance.

This passage expresses beautifully four things:

1. an intimate involvement with Yin and Yang

2. a removal from the 'common world'

3. an ability to store or 'build up' a purity which led to clear thinking

4. lastly, after a period of 'wandering', a return to the world of people.

It is through aping the bendability of the *yinyang* that we see the transitoriness of thought and reach a quiet beyond. An understanding of how Yin and Yang work in the mind allows an intuitive grasp of each and every situation. We tap into a natural wisdom. The reasoning of the School of Yin and Yang was perfectly suited to the rationalist theory needed in the *Neijing*. Later on, I will show how such a flexible, organic logic, founded upon the bedrock of the 'equality of all things', keeps us, better than any other method, in touch with the world.

In this initial discussion of Yin and Yang I simply want to illustrate how this subtle way of thought, born during the Warring States and Han, shows off the mind to its best advantage. The tale above of the ancient 'Adepts' hints that when using this tool in medicine one needs also to lay claim to an inner silence or quiet – a pensive time to develop one's own determination and faith – in order to put the *yinyang* and *wuxing* in order, and then subsequently carry out the medical task most fitting.

In the first few pages of *Suwen* 1 the physician Qi Bo describes 'detachment and peace, remaining humble and empty' in order to live well. Again, in the opening sentence to *Suwen* 17, in his discussion on pulse diagnosis, we are told there is 'an art in attending to the pulse – be humbled, quiet and guarded'. In *Suwen* 26 the finest physician is 'alert to the minutest of changes', and the same chapter, speaking of the 'clear mind' 神明 *shenming* or 'bright spirit', states:

> …the spirit is the spirit! Your ears cannot hear it. But when the eyes are bright and the heart opened, then your feelings come forward – quick and alert, and you are aware of it. But you alone understand. You cannot talk about it. Everyone looks for it, but only you see. Suddenly, from being in the dark, there comes a light. But it is a light for you, independently. It is like when the wind blows away the clouds. That is what we call the 'spirit'.

If you want to pursue this matter further you need to turn to the diagrams and trigrams in Appendix A. As the *Neijing* says, 'it is a light for you, independently'. It is not easy to communicate this inner silence and space in which the growth of Yin and Yang take place. Well, let the last word go to Xue Shengbai, commenting on the first chapter of Li Zhongzi's book, which had just been reprinted:

> What has been extracted here has not variously or carelessly been done, but is the business of 'guarding the one'… It is not honouring any other aspect but the 'three strangers' – the Tao, the Yin and the Yang. Generally speaking, if you view the pathway of the heavens above and keep a grasp on its cycle, you will advance your years to one hundred, along with the age-old ways of honouring life! They are the greatest! But truly to rely on a knowledge which is not founded on a sense of 'humility and inner peace' is to practise the evil arts. It is not to come back to the 'easy and simple' but only to be exploring its byways.

4. Li Zhongzi, His Compilation and the Quietly Enquiring Mind

There is a tale told of Li Zhongzi's encounter with the physician Wang Kentang, famous writer and populariser of medicine among the Ming middle classes – and certainly a figure senior to Li Zhongzi:

> When Wang Kentang was eighty years old he suffered diarrhoea caused by a deficiency in the spleen. All the company of doctors were concerned about his great age and failing body and immediately offered strengthening medicines – but the disease got worse and became troublesome. Li Zhongzi observed this and said: 'This gentleman's body is overweight, with too much phlegm. To heal and strengthen him, treat the obstruction. You should use a swiftly working, enabling medicine to scour the trouble out. Do not doubt what I say!' Now Kentang was also a skilled physician. He said: 'In the world of medicine, there are only two figures. The master here says: "This is the prescription", and I swallow it down! How can I doubt what he says?' Li Zhongzi then made up a crystalline powder out of the croton bean, in order to purge out the phlegm. There streamed out several pints of matter and Kentang was cured.

Now the croton bean is extremely toxic and a drastic purgative – and Li took great risks in using this prescription. He opposed the consensus of the doctors present, who would have used gentler tonics. But these were difficult times in this densely populated area of China. The bubonic plague ravaged the district in the spring of 1641; indeed, in the same year as Li's *Cornerstone* arrived, a *Treatise on Pestilence* was written and published by Wu Youxing. When the plague reached Peking the very next year it caused over 200, 000 deaths. It is sobering to think that the capitals of Europe were also falling at this time. Apothecaries and herbalists, east and west, were facing similar obstacles to their trade.

This was the year before the fall of the Ming, when the Manchus, first asked into Beijing to help subdue the rebels, finally took power and the last Ming emperor hanged himself. It was a time of great rebellion and political and social turmoil – and it was during these years that Dr Li produced his *Cornerstone*. There was undoubtedly a need for trained medical personnel at all levels of society, and the practicality of the book was paramount.

There had been abstracts of the *Neijing* before. Towards the end of the Yuan dynasty (1260–1368), Hua Shou devised his *Du Su Wen Chao, Copied-out Passages from the Su Wen*, which may be said to be the true forerunner to Li Zhongzi's selection. Hua Shou divided up the contents of the old medical books into 12 chapters, each covering a separate category of medical thought: (1) conditions of the internal organs, (2) dimensions of the channels, (3) pulse diagnosis, (4) pathology, (5) hygiene, (6) treatment, (7) complexion and pulse, (8) acupuncture, (9) Yin and Yang, (10) outer indications and inner causes, (11) cycles of the qi, and (12) summary of important points.

Then, some 300 years later, in 1624, Zhang Jiebin, a native of Zhejiang Province, compiled his *Lei Jing* or *Classifying the Classic*. This book, a colossal undertaking – and the work of a philological saint – took some 30 years, and was undertaken in the spirit of the Han learning which gained precedence during the later Qing dynasty. The idea was to recapture the original intention of the Han and return immediacy to medicine. Both Zhang and Li were pioneers in moving medical practice away from the grasp of Song and Yuan theorists, and giving it new life.

Zhang Jiebin was some 25 years older than Li Zhongzi and, since he lived and worked in neighbouring Zhejiang, the influence of the older man upon the younger is likely; especially so, in view of the fact that Li includes sections of Zhang's work verbatim in his commentary. It is worth noting that many famous Ming doctors were born in Jiangsu, Li Zhongzi's birthplace – Xue Ji, whom Li quotes, Wang Kentang the populariser (see the story above), Wu Youxing and Miao Xiyong, as well as Li Zhongzi himself. This prosperous coastal region now incorporates the large cities of Nanjing and Shanghai.

Zhang Jiebin ordered his texts slightly differently to Hua Shou: (1) Nurturing Health (hygiene), (2) Yin and Yang, (3) Zang Imagery (conditions of the *zang* organs), (4) Pulse and Colour (facial complexion), (5) The Jingluo (the energetic channels), (6) Branch and Root (outer indications and inner causes), (7) Qi and Taste (energetics of diet), (8) Discussion on Treatment, (9) Pathology, (10) Acupuncture Needling, (11) Cycles of the Energies (cycles of qi) and (12) Summary.

And Li's approach was different again to Zhang's. Li Zhongzi was a working physician and could not afford 30 years of secluded study. A feature of the *Cornerstone* is its distinctly practical nature. It was a book for beginners, readable by students. Li discarded more vacuous theorising – especially that inserted by Wang Bing during the Tang. He emphasised a quietly enquiring mind, a close examination of the patient and great sensitivity. One's practice had to be rooted in a feeling of 'utter humility and deep sense of peace' – a point he makes early in the book. Two extracts from his commentary illustrate this:

To reach for utter humility and deep sense of peace is to be 'guarding an emptiness' within. When all in the world receive an injury it is because of fullness and complacency. Join your body with the Void and you are never subject to baseness. Your life and destiny are inexhaustible and you end your days, along with the skies and the earth.

In cutting into the beat of the pulse, you are examining Yin and Yang; in looking at the brightness in the eyes, you are examining the mental strength. Observe the colours in the face and you may observe the weakness or strength of their organs; inspect the physical form of the body and you can separate out whether the sickness is filling or retreating. Take these several methods and contrast and combine them along with the picture of the pulse, in order to reach a conclusion. Then Yin and Yang, inner and outer, weakness and strength, cold and heat, are clearly visible and you may truly decide their lot of life and death.

Li Zhongzi's description of a quietly enquiring mind is typically Chinese. An understanding of the logic it involves will occupy us later. However, it can be glimpsed in an endearing poem which heads up his book *How to Stay Well without Medicines*, a compendium of writings on Taoist Yoga put together after his death.

> I have one small slab, a Magical Elixir,
> It can cure all errors throughout the Four Seas.
> Even a little child swallowing it, he settles,
> As it controls old age and puts a brake on destiny.
> Anyone may understand this core method of settling the heart,
> But it is without form, this mysterious medicine.
> If a doctor understands it he will never fall sick,
> He turns over his body to leap into the Great Void!
> Tangled thoughts from karmic retribution are many,
> All unsettled and disturbed! How to describe them…?
> Man with a cluttered mind displays thinking,
> But a thought without a cluttered mind, starts to produce Man.
> When Man's mind is uncluttered, it is vast, beyond thought;
> Ending thought – suddenly your sight gains great clarity!
> Here then becomes the same as over there.
> All is powdered, smashed up into dust!
> You begin to see a light…
> The clouds open and a thousand miles, a pathway is clear,
> The bright moon gleaming, round, pure, glistening and white…
> As I roam the Four Seas my care for life is inexhaustible –
> My heart joins with the jade-green waters, they join with the sky.
> At the ferry head, white-haired, an old fisherman questions me…
> Each day I understand, the peach blossoms, freshly born anew.

> From an inscription at *Forest Mirror Hall* Temple

Couched in this ornate language is an emphasis on the daily renewal of the innocent heart ('peach blossoms'), out of an uncluttered mind. Certainly Li Zhongzi saw an uncluttered mind as paramount. During these tumultuous times, a doctor had to keep a certain detachment about himself and Li saw this as preserving a Buddhist inner quiet.

Li Zhongzi's selections were chosen to illustrate the 'key' or 'cornerstone' to the work: the dynamic spring of the *yinyang* and *wuxing*, the interplay of seasonal change, the need for quiet in the mind, the primacy of the Yang, the careful scrutiny of each and every medical situation, and so on. He pointedly discarded the 'cycling of the qi' 運氣 *yunqi* chapters, inserted by later editors, and made use of only eight out of twelve headings used by his teacher Zhang Jiebin. Here are Li Zhongzi's chapters:

1. Ways of Life

2. Yin and Yang

3. Examination of the Complexion

4. Examination of the Pulse

5. The Zang Images

6. The Jingluo (Channels and Collaterals)

7. Rules in Treatment

8. Pathology

I have followed Li Zhongzi's categorisation, as I found it full of meaning. But I have also amended it slightly, and added other texts from the *Neijing* on the art and spirit of needling, on the origins of *wuxing* science and personality types, and lastly on 'faults and failings'.

To understand Li Zhongzi's particularly contemporary approach, we need to explore the thought of his period. During the late Ming the prevailing philosophical climate was still Confucian, but a Confucianism which embraced large 'chunks' of Taoism and Buddhism. One of its most seminal thinkers was Wang Yangming (1472–1529), doyen of the 'syncretist' school, which took the premise that *li* 理, literally 'the grain on wood' but, by extension, also 'pattern' or 'universal principle' – a term coined back in the

12th century – actually underpinned the whole world. Not only that, they also maintained that *li* operates *within us* as well as *through* the human mind. They understood the mind (or heart) to be made up of exactly 'the same stuff' as the world. Mind and world were close partners. As the Han would have it – 'heaven and man are one', governed by the 'Way' 道 *dao* (Tao). And how could this not be, since we are all part of nature? It follows, then, that to investigate the world we may as well investigate ourselves! Wang Yangming urges the removal of all selfish desires and prejudices from the person in order to see things clearly – and discover, at the same time, the original state of our knowing within (one might call it Buddha-nature, in all but name).

> The mind of man constitutes heaven in all its profundity, within which there is nothing not included. Originally there was nothing but this single heaven, but because of barriers caused by selfish desire, we have lost this original state of heaven. If we now concentrate our thoughts upon extending our intuitive knowledge, so as to sweep away all barriers and obstructions, the original state will then again be restored, and we will again become part of the profundity of heaven.

This is how Confucianism became 'idealistic' during the Ming, largely under the influence of Yangming. The influence of Buddhism, especially Chan Buddhism (Zen), is evident. Again Wang Yangming states:

> When I speak about the extension of knowledge through the investigation of things, I mean by this an extension of our mind's intuitive knowledge into all affairs and things. This intuitive knowledge of our mind is what is known as Heavenly Principle (天理 *tian li*).

Yangming takes the phrase 'the extension of knowledge through the investigation of things' 致知在格物 *zhi zhi zai ge wu* from the opening paragraphs of the Confucian text, the *Great Learning*.

His mention of an 'intuitive knowledge' 良知 *liang zhi* again stems from the thinker Mencius.

> When I speak about the extension of knowledge through the investigation of things, I mean by this an extension of our mind's intuitive knowledge into all affairs and things. This intuitive knowledge of our mind is also what is known as Heavenly Principle (*tian li*).

The catchphrase 'the investigation of things' 格物 *gewu* is often quoted by Chinese scholars. For Yangming it was simply self-evident that following the work of extending the mind's intuitive knowledge was the same as representing *li*.

The commentary to the initial hexagram 'Creation' (1) in the Imperial Qing edition of the *Yijing* (the *Zhouyi Zhezhong*, published in 1715) follows the same line; giving precedence to *li*:

> As life first is created, it manifests as a Grand Harmony within primordial chaos. This is the source. As energy stirs, a pattern (*li*) is disclosed: thus the source provides for blessings. Then it assumes form as principle (*li*) within the heart, as our self-nature – and so that which is blessed attains a favoured course throughout the world. The Grand Harmony is preserved and all unified, attaining its ultimate goal in human devotion.

I will have more to say about *li* and intuitive knowledge later, when I discuss the boundaries of Chinese thought.

Li Zhongzi wanted to show that in medicine the craft, the art and the science are all one. This was directly in line with Yangming's thinking. For Yangming the deep mind is the true goal of our study – not accumulated learning or an ability to argue. This dependence on one's own innermost commitment to any situation represented the independent spirit of the Ming. They believed that true creativity came from the heart and should not be tainted by too much learning. Perhaps it was an increased frustration at the social and political world around them.

Li Zhongzi also understood that the goal of medical training must sometimes be discreet and plainly simple. If we can realise our innate nature, our original 'good heart', we may find completion, inner peace and certitude – and, at the same time, be able wholly to apply ourselves to the task at hand. Henceforth, such a doctor would act, not solely in line with theory or book learning, 'fame or profit', but also as one human being facing another, concerned over their suffering and treating all kindly – as members of his or her own immediate family. This was in good accord with Confucian ethics.

5. A World Refracted through Chinese Language

I have given the original texts from the *Neijing* – as we need to delve into the Chinese language in order to fully understand Chinese medicine. What is it in the nature of the Chinese script that gives it such intrigue? That makes it, at once, so baffling and yet full of fascination for the Western scholar? Understanding Chinese script demands an appreciation of how it works. Ways of language reflect ways of thought. Chinese differs radically from Indo-European – including English, or French, for that matter – for the Chinese pictorial characters (not letters) were first and foremost *drawn from life*, not recorded sounds.

This means that a written shape was a direct visual representation or picture of a situation. For example, the English written word 'sun', or 'man' (or French '*soleil*', or '*homme*'), is a direct phonetic record of the spoken word. But in Chinese the character for 'sun' 日 (just a square with a line in it, showing a point of light), or 'man' 人 (the two legs are obvious), existed prior to any need for speech. A page of classical characters (which have no tense, no person, no number) demands involvement of a greater part of the brain, just as does a French pointillist painting, an Elizabethan sonnet, a Bach fugue or a complex algebraic formula. The Chinese mind is not so easily encouraged into mental discrimination. Both Indian and European cultures have a Graeco-Roman alphabet based upon phonemes, or the smallest units of sound in a language. But in China, the picture came first – and it remains so.

The Chinese language is therefore primarily visual, therefore *closer to nature*, and more involved in the here-and-now, fist-hittable world. It does not so easily encourage the distractions and abstractions which Westerners slip into, with their composite 'words' and 'concepts' made of symphonies of sounds. Pictures allow a deeper grasp of the physical structure of any situation.

Cheng Chung-ying, one-time Professor of Philosophy at the University of Hawaii, states:

> As a phonetic language, the Greek language is auditorily orientated and tends to present a world of meanings in separation from a world of concrete things. For there is nothing in the phonetic symbols of the Greek language to suggest the presence of sensible objects. This easily leads to conceptual abstractions, certainly more easily than would an image-language such as the Chinese language. The separation of the sensible from the non-sensible can thus become an inherent tendency in the use of a phonetic language just as the cohesion of the sensible with the non-sensible can become a fundamental feature of the use of an image-language.

In other words, the sensible is intrinsic to Chinese thought. Chinese pictograms – much, much more so than letters in an alphabet – point to a physical world. Perhaps more importantly, Western thinking, especially that schooled in texts without oral instruction or apprenticeship, traps sensory experience in *concepts*, hampering further thought and, more crucially, further perception. Cheng continues:

> …the Greek language, being a phonetic language, produces an abstraction of thinking more easily than the visual language of Chinese. This tendency toward abstraction is conducive to transcendental thinking in extensive abstractions and thus leads to the crystallization of both thinking and the object of

thinking in an enclosure of concepts. The Chinese language, however, being rooted in the concrete representation of the reality of experience orientated both visually and auditorily, always brings the image of the world to metaphysical contemplation.

In other words, the Chinese think more in pictures, closer to the concrete. In his introduction to an excellent set of Chinese-language primers, the American sinologist and teacher H. G. Creel makes the point that:

> literary Chinese…is not 'writing' in the sense that written English is 'writing'. That is, it is not a recording of speech. It consists, instead, of a series of suggestive idea-centres (characters) which vary in their content and in their relation to each other, depending upon the total context, as constantly and as unpredictably as light on rippling water…consequently the reading of literary Chinese is a creative, not a passive, task.

Are these shifting 'idea-centres', identity and difference (Yin and Yang), and their unpredictability of outcome perhaps a true analogue of the way the mind (or human brain) works? I believe they mimic the on/off firing of the neurons and their changing electrical charge, which we interpret as Yin (negative) and Yang (positive). This is another argument for associationism, which sees linking ideas to be the basis of all mental processes. Is it any wonder then that classical Chinese encourages such fast-moving and flexible thinking? Images, like pictures, subtly bend and change. They involve humour, drama and play, and are closer to experience. Imaginative thinking is actually more demanding. It is more childlike – it always seems to want more! The Chinese language is pictorial, laconic and unwordy. It uses poetical associations. Why is this? Because images mean there is no gap in communication; they are more true-moving, and full of vitality – like life itself! Listen to Wang Bi (3rd century), a brilliant young mind, as he speaks about words, imaginative thinking and meaning in his essay on the *Yijing*:

> Imaginative thinking (*xiang*) serves to express the meaning (*yi*); while words (*yan*, literally 'spoken words', or even text) serve to explain imaginative thinking. For the complete expression of meaning there is nothing like imaginative thinking, and for the complete explanation of imaginative thinking, there is nothing like the words. Words are generated by images, so by pondering the words one may perceive the images. Images are generated by meaning, so by pondering the images one may perceive the meaning. The meaning is completely expressed by the imaginative thinking and the images completely explained by the words. Therefore since the purpose of the words is to explain the images, once the images have been grasped, the words may be forgotten. And since the purpose of the images is to preserve the meaning, once the meaning has been grasped, the images may be forgotten... Similarly, as Zhuangzi said, 'the snare exists for the rabbit – once you have caught the rabbit, you can forget the snare! And the fish-trap exists for the fish, so once you get the fish, you can forget the trap!' This being so, the words act as a snare for the imagination and the imagination is a trap for the meaning.

In this compact passage, Wang Bi shows that clinging to imaginative thinking, or a text, or spoken words, and not seeing them in dynamic relationship to each other, takes the life out of them. They no longer work as they should. It is the dynamic *yinyang* in the pictogram – pointing to the concrete world – that stimulates the imaginative thinking which so epitomises the Chinese character and, *a fortiori*, supplies both depth and flexibility to the Chinese mind. Chinese language approaches closer to nature. It demands involvement in depth; and becomes self-referential, which is the distinction of all poetry.

It is all very simple. We need to trust our senses and innermost feelings to be truly human – as well as to make intellectual

ᴐ

)ns, to observe, carefully and meticulously, the world
In the chapter on facial diagnosis it is the observable light
.ty of the face which is most important. The quality of the
'sɪᴄᴋ pulse is 'rough, tough and hard' – not soft. This is something
we feel. But if we are not open to our senses, we will not feel or
understand it. The distinction between hard and soft also occurs
in the Taoist volume, the *Laozi* (76):

> The stiff and unyielding is the disciple of death,
> While the soft and yielding is the disciple of life.

Again consider these phrases from the chapter on patterns in
treatment, where common, practical sense comes to the fore:

> If they are cold, then heat them.
> If they are hot, then cool them down.
> If the condition is slight, you can work against it.
> If it is severe, then go along with it.

This reflects a 'no-nonsense' attitude possessed by a down-to-earth
people. Perhaps it derives from a life lived closer to agricultural
and rural roots. An appreciation of the 'concrete', founded in these
texts, will hopefully re-ground the present practice of Chinese
medicine; returning it to *li*, or at least something close to it.

6. Claude Levi-Strauss and the Untamed Mind

The French social anthropologist Claude Levi-Strauss (1908–
2009) has done much to help towards an understanding of
the deeper and more 'primitive' structures of the brain, as they
function on the level of sensation (that is, beyond words). I would
like to introduce some of his ideas to illustrate again the bifocal
nature of the *yinyang*.

Levi-Strauss uncovered the structure of primitive thought in
his enormously erudite book *The Savage Mind*. In this book he
indicates that peculiarly sensory-orientated mode of thought in

'primitives', born in what he calls the 'savage mind'. Yet his ideas have broadly influenced our modern appreciation of how thinking works – that is, the structuralist approach to all human activity and phenomena, which, put rather too simply, says that we really only understand through looking at interrelations. And although I do not follow Levi-Strauss's erudite analysis and conclusion entirely, his train of thought is clear. He describes two distinctive modes of scientific enquiry – two distinct ways in which nature may be accessible to human thought:

> ...two strategic levels at which nature is accessible to scientific enquiry: one roughly adapted to that of perception and the imagination; the other at a remove from it...two different routes, one very close to, and the other more remote from, sensible intuition.

His quest for a universal underlying structure within the human mind strays close to Wang Yangming's assertion that 'principle' or 'patterning' underpins all human thinking. However, one difference is that in Yangming the mind, freed of its patent desires, will become identical with Heaven's true pattern. Yangming's characteristically moral implication is that it is *selflessness* which enables us to gain the true path, the path of self-development and clear understanding.

Levi-Strauss likewise believed that there were underlying patterns of thought involved in all human discourse and activity. This view reached its full fruit in his massive and impressive four-volume *Mythologiques I, II, III, IV*. In these works he puts his finger accurately on the mind's different functions of creating unity and separation. His analysis within this grand edifice is built on the two functions of *identity* and *difference*. Put simply, his argument is that mankind reacted to the mystery of the world by inventing myths to explain it: for example, how we discovered fire, how the edible and inedible came into being, how the celestial and terrestrial, the human and animal, are interrelated, and so on. This develops into a thought which had the distinction of being 'concrete' – in that its logic was constructed out of observable contrasts in the sensory qualities of 'things'; that is, hard and soft, wet and dry, light and dark, high and low, and, by extension, the skies and earth, man and woman, and so on – and also that this was put together by picking up what was around us, from a richer, natural world.

Interestingly enough, I have thought for years that the mind (with its ideas and concepts) often seeks to work like a 'bodger' – patching up the world, and giving meaning to our somewhat chaotic lives. Traditionally a bodger was one who lived in the forest and turned wood for a trade, using a pole-lathe, but more recently it has been taken to mean one who acquires useful materials, practically anything to hand, in order to finish a task. The result may not always be predictable, pretty or elegant, but it is fit for purpose. The mind is always working towards a solution. Levi-Strauss also compared the activity of the 'primitive' mind to that of a *'bricoleur'* (French 'handyman'). Perhaps we might call him a DIY enthusiast, going about his task, making do with whatever he can find.

It is hard not to see the *yinyang* as a complete description of this process: a light, moving organism pitted against a dark, fairly inert environment. Yin and Yang are *dynamic in nature*. This is the very point of the wavy line dividing them. To miss this is to miss the nature of life. In small scale, they show the on–off firing of the synapses in the brain, or the struggling interface between inner and outer at the cell wall, the sodium–potassium pump essential for neural communication; in large scale, the reciprocating activity of the immune response, the boundary between self and other – the reaction that wards off an attack. Yin and Yang give us perspective, order and meaning. They allow us a place to breathe.

Of course this so-called 'primitive' mode of *yinyang* thinking is not primitive at all – a fact which Levi-Strauss certainly appreciated. Rather it is that form of thought closest to the physical world – closest to organic and biological form. What he calls 'sensible intuition' is actually the most immediate thought of dreams, fables and fiction. It is interesting to note that even the

English anthropologist Radcliffe-Brown, to whom Levi-Strauss owed much, turned to these ideas just before his death. In his last paper Radcliffe-Brown spoke of 'that association by contrariety that is a universal feature of human thinking, so that we think by pairs of contraries, upwards and downwards, strong and weak, black and white'.

This development of 'binary oppositions' through Levi-Strauss's vast investigation of primitive myth provides an excellent example of the *yinyang* in action. He would also contend that there is no break between so-called 'primitive' and more sophisticated methods of reasoning. Both operate under an implicit logic, which can truly only be understood as it is seen working.

7. A Logic of Tangible Qualities

Levi-Strauss coined the phrase 'a logic of tangible qualities' to describe this logic of the concrete. This is distinct from the logic of abstractions – common in Western scientific thinking. In the introduction to *The Raw and the Cooked: Introduction to a Science of Mythology I*, he states: 'The aim of this book is to show how empirical categories – such as the categories of the raw and the cooked, the fresh and the decayed, the moistened and the burned, etc. can be used as conceptual tools with which to elaborate abstract ideas and combine them in the form of propositions. ' He also wants to prove the common significance of this logic of the senses – which apprehends the real world.

In the *Mythologiques* Levi-Strauss is able to reveal how *yinyang* structures create human thinking. He demonstrates a systematic ordering behind human expression, involving the senses. He shows that single cultural terms in a system can only be properly understood *in relationship* to other elements of that same system, and that each system is built up through contrasts or oppositions (Yin and Yang), which in turn reveal the innate structuring of the human mind.

This is where we come back to *li*. Think of *li* as complementary to qi; a feeling for the underlying make-up of things. In the appendices to the *Yijing* (*Book of Change*) it is stated: 'What is *before form* may be called the Way; what is *after form* may be called the utensil.' Let me try to explain – the shape of a leaf, the ripples on water, the sound of an axe chopping wood in the distance, or a dog barking – all these are certainly evidence of *li*. *Li* can play Yin to qi's Yang. Perhaps we could call *li* the 'grain' of the work. That which is 'before form' is something other – that which is 'after form' is the 'utensil' – in other words, it is put to use in the physical world. Here we are talking about spirit in matter. To reveal the underlying pattern has been my intent in presenting these medical texts. Whether this pattern is expressed as *yinyang*, *wuxing* or *li* is practically irrelevant.

Remember Li Zhongzi's poem from *Forest Mirror Hall*?

Man with a cluttered mind displays thinking,
But a thought, without a cluttered mind, starts to produce Man.
When Man's mind becomes uncluttered, it is vast, beyond
    thought –
Ending thought – suddenly your sight gains great clarity!

This is a perception of the patterning of *li*. The *yinyang* function displays both integration and separation, synthesis and analysis. When 'a cluttered mind displays thinking' – we have analysis and differentiation; when 'thought, without a cluttered mind' appears, it suggests feeling, intuition and synthesis. The Chinese mind is no more than a fuller mind, a mind of the concrete – as well as a mind of abstractions. A true medical science involves both, but *primarily* an in-depth investigation into each and every clinical situation. This is what we might call the 'before-form'. No patient ever presents the same way twice. But noticing this is only possible when one is educated in depth – yes, through book learning, but also through oral instruction, demonstration, failure and world experience. It is the clinical skills that are most striking in a doctor, for therein lies the craft. Herein lies the seed of self-scrutiny, doubt, moral plenitude and integrity so characteristically Confucian.

Mencius believed that man's nature need only to be blended with good form or 'propriety' to become *jen* ('love, kindness'). This escapes the moral imperatives so dear to Western hearts, the 'thou shalt' and 'shalt not's of the Ten Commandments. In contradistinction to Christian ethics, the Chinese moral ideal was a mixing of inward nature with outer harmony, a harmony both social and universal. Out of this blend came our innate goodness, which meant to be helpful in the long run by 'making the people anew'. Goodness comes about naturally, through self-cultivation. It is not to be emulated in itself, but rather arises as we devote ourselves towards self-scrutiny and a committed investigation of the world. Levi-Strauss aimed to reveal the structure of primitive thought, the 'soft underbelly' of modern thinking. Although working within the confines of the Académie Française, he was able to show how individual elements within a system can only be properly understood in relation to other elements of that system, and how each system is built up through contrasts or oppositions which reveal the innate functioning of the human mind. The relevance to the *yinyang* tool is obvious.

Chinese medical thinking, in fact all Chinese thinking, centres on *relation* and *process* – it is not usually end-centred. It encourages patterning, an appreciation of the sensory world, and a touch which is quite special. Professor Kuang-ming Wu has said:

> Chinese medicine is pattern-thinking, phenomena-discerning, and takes things as interpenetrative…if to understand something in Western medicine is to grasp bodily parts and causes linearly and quantitatively, then to understand a phenomenon in Chinese medicine is to discern patterns of bodily dynamism in the environment uniquely and coordinately. Such discernment has the touch of the painter going from a simple drawing to a fine painting.

Chinese medicine in thinking and sensing involves 'deep' structure. It is aided by the dual activity of the mind, building up a total picture of each situation: at once analytic, and *at the same time* synthetic and unitary. Compare, for example, the poetic pulse qualities given in *Suwen* 17:

> On spring days the pulse is 'floating',
> Like a fish suspended in the eddy of a stream;
> On summer days the pulse lies at the skin,
> Floating freely, everything in surplus.
> On autumn days it lies under the skin,
> Like a torpid insect ready to creep away.
> On winter days it lies at the bone,
> Like a torpid insect, totally hidden –

Last, let us look again at the characters of the internal organs of the body given in *Suwen* 5:

> The heart is the office of the lord and master. A clear mind is his duty. The lungs are the officials of communications. Government and regulation are their duty. The liver is the official of the military commander. Plotting and planning are his duty. The gallbladder is the official of inner integrity. Making decisions and judgements is his duty.

This is certainly poetry. The organs of the human body are given personalities and characters. A concrete logic such as this means that right action is all-important. It matters not that such-and-such concept fits with such-and-such concept to form a pattern of thought – rather, the issues are: 'Does it work here?' 'Does it ring true?' 'Will I get the patient well?' Appropriate action, that which works, is paramount. It is difficult for a Western mind to understand the Confucian emphasis on 'propriety' 禮 *li*, the second of their four grand virtues – for he or she is looking to see if any particular situation fits into any previously thought-out framework. What is at issue is not a mechanistic view of the world, but a theory of organism.

The idea of healthy living and appropriate treatment outlined in Li Zhongzi's *Cornerstone* meant a resonance with the thought processes of the *yinyang* and *wuxing*, or the natural, seasonal pattern of 'birth and growth, closure and storage' 生長, 收藏 *shengzhang, shouzang*. Such a resonance encouraged harmony and health in both the patient and the doctor, and enabled them to decide upon any treatment which would restore and maintain harmony.

8. Conclusion: A Divide in Medical Thinking

In China, ever since the turn of the 19th century, at the collapse of the Qing dynasty and the establishment of the Republic in 1912, a new language, and new thinking – influenced greatly by the West – evolved in that country. It emerged out of the remnants of the logic of tangible qualities of old, and it is this language that determines how Chinese medicine is understood and taught at present in China, and also predominantly in the West.

But Chinese medicine incorporates more than an enquiring intellect: it is not only interested in what is being said – but also in the who, the why, the how, the when, the to-whom and the wherefore. It is not so determinedly end-centred, as are the more rigidly structured chains of reasoning in Aristotelian logic. It is inclusive, sounding out an appreciation of *any aspect* of a situation, and has a quite unique sensitivity to many correlates. In its fluidity and depth, and physical involvement in the 'right now', it involves a combination of seeing, sensing and thinking which is peculiarly Chinese.

It is this depth of perception and commitment to a theory of organism which made the Chinese such natural scholars. Joseph Needham says at the conclusion of his discussion on 'spagyria and alchemy':

> The key-word in the old Chinese thought-system was order, but this was an order based on organic pattern, and indeed on a hierarchy of organisms. The symbolic correlations or correspondences all formed part of one colossal pattern. Things behaved in particular ways not necessarily because of prior action or chance impulsions of other things, but because their position in the ever-moving cyclical universe was such that they were endowed with intrinsic natures which made that

behaviour inevitable for them. If they did not behave in those particular ways they would lose their relational positions in the whole which made them what they were, and turn into something other than themselves. They were thus organic parts in existential dependence upon the whole world-organism, and they reacted upon one another not so much by mechanical impulse or causation as by a kind of mysterious resonance.

This resonance or 'mutual interaction', *xiangying*, lies at the core of the *Neijing*'s ideas about the 'arts and ways of a good life' outlined in the first chapters of the book, a resonance with the old rhythms of life, and a proper respect for both Yin and Yang – fundamental to their truths.

Let us leave the last word to Laozi: 'The ancients, who knew the truth, did not try to enlighten others. They kept them in the dark. Why are the people so difficult to heal? It is because they know too much. '

In other words, it takes an acquired knowledge to remove us from the truth. Over-thinking takes us away from the world in front of our noses, and leads us into tortuous chains of argument. It is the *yinyang*, the logic of tangible qualities, that keeps us in touch (literally) with, and alive to, the world. It is crucial practice for patient and practitioner alike and means both the preserve of our own good health and learning of how to heal.

These texts have been chanted and memorised by countless lips and tongues, now turned to dust. The Taoists would have it that our sojourn in this world is but a brief interlude in the great and grand passage of time: the mind-numbing darkness and bounty of space which peoples our universe. This book follows in the footsteps of many pioneers, notably Huang Fumi, Wang Bing, Zhang Jiebin, Li Zhongzi and Gia-fu Feng. This was the single idea – in the mind of the Yellow Emperor. One mind, one thought, one light, one dark, one people, one world. As the old Kings would have it, 'there is no separation in the land'.

Characters in the Introduction

the ancients 古 *gu*

love, kindness, human-heartedness 仁 *jen*

rightness in action 義 *yi*

a sense of propriety 禮 *li*

wisdom 智 *zhi*

heart, mind 心 *xin*

the emperor, supreme authority 帝 *di*

yinyang 陰陽 *yinyang*

wuxing 五行 *wuxing*

element or force 行 *xing*

mutual interaction 相应 *xiangying*

truly human, realised 真人 *zhenren*

clear mind, bright spirit 神明 *shenming*

cycling of the qi 運氣 *yunqi*

pattern, universal principle, the grain on wood 理 *li*

the Way, method, 'arts' 道 *dao*

Heavenly Principle 天理 *tian li*

the extension of knowledge through the investigation of things 致知在格物
    zhi zhi zai ge wu

intuitive knowledge 良知 *liang zhi*

the investigation of things 格物 *gewu*

birth and growth, closure and storage 生長, 收藏 *shengzhang, shouzang*

I

The Arts and Ways
of a Good Life

The Wise ones, their model lay in the skies and earth,
their imagination as the sun and moon, their discernment
akin to the full array of stars which reveal the time.

Key Ideas

1. *The Yellow Emperor Questions his Counsellor*
   antiquity, the Emperor's introduction, the regret over his people, Qi Bo's answer

2. *A Message from the Ancients*
   the ancient Sages, their teachings, the malign *xie*, the thief-wind, being at peace, the real qi, mental strength

3. *They Represented the Arts and Ways of Life*
   real substance, Yin and Yang, the breath, Adepts, Sages, the wise, longevity

4. *The Rhythm of the Seasons*
   spring–life; summer–abundance; autumn–closure; winter–storage; a seasonal response, the qi

5. *The Energy of the Yang Stored up*
   the heavenly qi, storage, the *yinyang*, failure, withering, the Sages

6. *The Practice of Advancing the Yang*
   the root of life and death, longevity, destiny

7. *Taoist Yoga*
   stilling the mind, stretching the neck, swallowing saliva

8. *The Sages Treated those Well, not those Sick*
   anticipation, early intervention

9. *The Character of the Malign Xie or Thief-Wind*
   the malicious climate, the eight winds

Some questions for review can be found at the end of this chapter.

1. The Yellow Emperor Questions his Counsellor

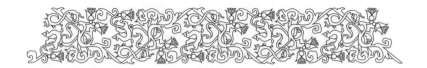

黃帝曰: 余聞上古之人, 春秋皆度百歲, 而動作不衰.
今時之人, 年半百而動作皆衰者, 時世異耶, 人將失之耶?

THE YELLOW EMPEROR ASKED:
I have heard it said that, in ancient times,
People's lives lasted a hundred springs and autumns,
And that they remained active and creative without getting old.
In the present age they reach fifty, half that number,
And they are already old –
What is different about our Age?
What is it the people have lost?

歧伯對曰: 上古之人, 其知道者, 法於陰陽, 和於術數.
食飲有節, 起居有常, 不妄作勞. 故能形與神俱, 而盡終其天年,
　　度百歲乃去.

Qi Bo replied: The people of old, they understood the Way,
They modelled themselves on the Yin and Yang
And were at peace with the arts of destiny.
Their eating and drinking were in moderation,
They rose and retired at regular hours,
They neither had wild ideas, nor wearied themselves out at work.
Thus they were able to keep body and soul together
And so attain the end of their natural span,
One hundred years and then pass away.

Wang Bing: The arts of destiny are no more than the great matter of preserving our lives. They who would care for themselves must diligently attend first to them.

今時之人不然也, 以酒為漿, 以妄為常.
醉以入房, 以欲竭其精, 以耗散其真.

The people of this age are not the same.
They drink liquor to excess,
And take wild ideas as the norm.
When drunk they perform the act of love,
Seeking to exhaust their qi and waste their true lives.

不知持滿, 不時御神, 務快其心, 逆於生樂.
起居無節, 故半百而衰也.

They do not know how to be content.
They have no time to control their thoughts,
Looking only for what cheers,
Not for the joys of health.
They rise and retire at any time –
And thus, at only fifty, are already weak.

At the opening of the *Neijing Suwen*, the main corpus of Chinese medical writings from Han times, the semi-mythical Yellow Emperor questions his medical counsellor. He asks why his people are not surviving into old age – as they did in ancient times. His medical advisor Qi Bo replies that it is because they have turned away from the ways of Yin and Yang, and neglected the 'arts of destiny'. These were the natural practices of preserving health, woven into a healthy lifestyle, simply following the rhythm of the seasons. During the Han, these skills were redefined in terms of the *yinyang* 陰陽 (Yin, Yang) and *wuxing* 五行 (Five Elements), and used, more generally, to influence, hurry along or turn aside misfortune. Medically the *yinyang* and *wuxing* were used to catalogue and understand the human body and mind, in all aspects of health and disease. They encouraged flexibility and depth of thought. This age saw the nascence of Chinese science, extracting itself from the exigencies of witchcraft and sorcery.

2. A Message
from the Ancients

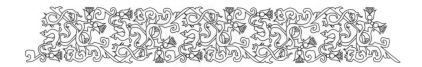

夫上古聖人之教下也, 皆謂之虛邪賊風. 避之有時.

NOW THE ANCIENT SAGES PROCLAIMED their teachings
  to the multitude, and they said:
There is such a thing as being weak and caught by the malign *xie*,
Or thieved by the wind.
Avoid it in time!

恬惔虛無, 真氣從之. 精神內守, 病安從來.

Be at peace, remain humble and empty,
And the real qi will follow.
The mental strength. Guard it within!
How then can sickness arrive?

Li Zhongzi: Being humble and empty signifies an 'utter humility and deep sense of peace'.

Wang Bing: The malign *xie* encroaches on the weakness and invades. This explains how when we are weak, we are caught by the *xie*. It stealthily destroys our inner harmony. This is why it is a 'thief-wind'.

Li Zhongzi: It is like a thief entering the room to rob us of what we have.

Zhang Jiebin: Feeling utterly deserted – one's heart is one's own, unmoved.

These first chapters in the *Neijing Suwen* introduce its view of the world. Fundamentally, it is contrived to be a record of the old teachings. The Han Chinese thought of themselves as heirs to a tradition of ancient Kings, the three 'mounds' (that is, burial mounds) of Fuxi, Shen Nong and Huangdi (the Yellow Emperor). It was Fuxi (the Subduer of Forms) who invented the symbols of the *Yijing* (*Book of Change*). Shen Nong (the Divine Husbandman) was the originator of herbal lore, while the Yellow Emperor instructed in the arts of medicine. Confucius, in his *Analects*, famously said, 'I am a transmitter, not an originator, I believe in and love the ancients. ' In *Suwen* 1 each of its several sections refers back to the 'ancient Sages' 古聖 *gusheng* and their teachings.

How is that we fall sick? The answer is that illness enters in from without to disturb our inner equilibrium. 'There is such a thing as being weak' – this describes a 'weak' 虚 *xu* or empty condition; while being caught by the 'malign' 邪 *xie* describes the invasion of a perverse or pathogenic factor, epitomised as climatic change or irregularity. The text continues to stress the state of ataraxy (imperturbability), and the cultivation of peace of mind. Not embracing an over-weaning strength enables the real qi 真氣 *zhen qi* to be born and to return. But then, if we keep strong – will we not fall? Not if our strength also embraces gentleness, humility and 'emptiness'. To be full invites decline. *Laozi* 19 says: 'Fill a cup to the brim and it will overflow, a blade over-sharpened cannot be kept long. ' This attitude stands at the heart of self-cultivation. The epitome of a humble self-care permeates both Taoist and Confucian ethics. Within a peaceful mind resides the natural breath. Again, *Laozi* 14 says: 'Watch…but it cannot be seen, it is so blurred. Listen…but it cannot be heard, it is so hushed. Grasp…but it cannot be held, it is so minute. ' The whole passage is in accord with the Taoist scriptures, which emphasise holding to the mind 精神 *jingshen* or 'mental strength', at the same time as softening the breath.

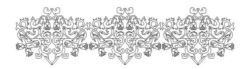

3. They Represented the Arts and Ways of Life

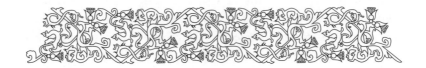

余聞上古有真人者. 提挈天地,
把握陰陽, 呼吸精氣, 獨立守神, 肌肉若一.

I HAVE HEARD IT SAID: In those times
There were people of real substance.
They lifted and raised up the skies and earth,
They grasped Yin and Yang in their own hands.
Their out-breath and in-breath were pure qi, as they stood alone,
    guarding the mind –
Their muscles and flesh as one.

故能壽敞天地, 無有終時, 此其道生.

Thus their longevity was able to wear out the skies and earth.
And being out of all time –
They represented the arts and ways of a good life.

Li Zhongzi: These people remained totally natural in their behaviour.

Zhang Jiebin: The art is of keeping to oneself – so that then one can stand alone.

Laozi: I acknowledge suffering because I acknowledge my own body. When I no longer have a body, how can I suffer!

有至人者, 淳德全道. 和于陰陽, 調于四時.
去世離俗, 積精全神. 游行天地之間, 視聽八遠之外.

And then there were the Adepts.
Lofty virtue reached its fulfilment in their curious ways.

They lived in peace with Yin and Yang,
And were in harmony with the four seasons.
They left the common world, away from all custom,
Building up a purity to fashion their minds in their entirety.
Travelling and wandering 'twixt the skies and earth,
They looked and listened
At all points of the compass.

此蓋益其壽命而強者也, 亦歸于真人.
Finally this promoted their longevity and destiny
And they became strong.
This returned them to being as people of real substance.

Li Zhongzi: Formerly the people of real substance represent the arts and ways of the good life. Now, in the case of the Adepts, longevity and destiny are mentioned, implying strength. But physical strength can only make the body whole – that is all. So they returned to being people of real substance which was as if they 'tempered the mind and returned it to the void' – for then they attained the same as the true people above. In this context, making the body whole through self-cultivation is the mark of the Adept.

其次有聖人者, 處天地之和, 從八風之理.
適嗜欲于世俗之間, 無恚嗔之心.
And then there were the Sagely ones,
Who resided at peace with the skies and earth,
Following the pattern of the 'eight winds'.
They fitted their likes and dislikes into worldly custom,
And had not the least resentment or craving in their hearts.

行不欲離于世, 被服章, 舉不欲觀于俗,
外不勞形於事, 內無思想之患.
In their behaviour they did not wish to be apart from the world;
While in their covering, ceremonial robes and decoration,
They served without needing to observe fashion.
Outwardly they were not over-busy with work,
While inwardly they avoided troubling thoughts or ideas.

以恬愉為務, 以自得為功.
形體不敝, 精神不散, 亦可以百數.

They made calm compassion their business
And self-contentment their task.
Their bodies were unworn, their minds uneroded,
And thus they were able to live out their hundred years!

Li Zhongzi: The Sages of old possessed a greatness and yet transcended it, for they surpassed all categorisation in human terms.

其次有賢人者, 法則天地, 象似日月, 辨列星辰.
逆從陰陽, 分別四時.
Lastly there were the Wise ones.
Their model lay in the skies and earth,
As images they had the sun and moon,
Their discernment akin to the full array of stars which reveal the
     time.
They acted in accordance with Yin and Yang,
And separated out and recognised the distinction between the
     four seasons.

Zhang Jiebin: Next to the Adepts come the wise. The Wise ones excel. They may be called the truly talented.

將從上古合同于道, 亦可使益壽而有極時.
Acting and following these people of ancient times,
You may unite together on the path.
Likewise you further increase your time on this earth,
And reach the fullness of your years.

This section describes, in orderly fashion, the ideal people of old, who were whole and healthy in body and mind. The 'people of real substance' 真人 *zhen ren* (more spiritual), the Adepts 至人 *zhi ren* (more worldly and practical), the Sages 聖人 *sheng ren* (detached from the world) and the Wise ones 賢人 *xian ren* (talented and more attached) are mentioned. The wise could be those working as physicians. Four classes of people are listed – but all deserve due mention for the honour and attention they give to the preservation of life. For the 'eight winds' see 'The Character of the Malign *Xie* or Thief-Wind', the final section of this chapter.

EULOGY ON HUMANKIND

People of real substance	lifted and raised up the skies and earth	grasped Yin and Yang in their own hands	out-breath and in-breath were pure qi	they stood alone, guarding the mind	their muscles and flesh as one	their longevity was able to wear out the skies and earth
Adepts	their lofty virtue reached fulfilment in their curious ways	lived in peace with Yin and Yang	were in harmony with the four seasons	left the common world, away from all custom, building up a purity to fashion their minds	wandering 'twixt the skies and earth, they looked and listened at all points of the compass	this promoted their longevity and destiny and they became strong
Sagely ones	they resided at peace with the skies and earth	following the pattern of the 'eight winds'	fitted their likes and dislikes into worldly custom, without the least resentment or craving in their hearts	did not wish to be apart from the world, in their covering, ceremonial robes and decoration, they served without needing to observe fashion	not over-busy with work, inwardly they avoided troubling ideas, they made calm compassion their business and self-contentment their task	their bodies unworn, their minds uneroded, they were thus able to live out their hundred years
Wise ones	their model lay in the skies and earth	as images they had the sun and moon	their discernment akin to the full array of stars which reveal the time	acted in accordance with Yin and Yang	separated out and recognised the distinction between the four seasons	following these people of ancient times, you unite with them on the path, to reach the fullness of your years

4. The Rhythm of the Seasons

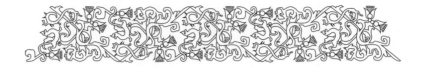

春三月, 此為發陳.

IN SPRINGTIME THERE ARE THREE MOONS,
This is a time for breaking out and bursting.

天地俱生, 萬物以榮.
夜臥早起, 廣步于庭, 被髮緩形, 以使志生,
生而勿殺, 予而勿奪, 賞而勿罰.
此春氣之應, 養生之道也.

The skies and the earth both give birth and all myriad creatures
    prosper.
Go to sleep at nightfall and rise at dawn.
Take large steps out in the courtyard.
Uncoil your hair and stretch out the body, thus to set the will on
    birth.
Help bring forth life and do not slaughter,
Help donate and do not take away,
Help reward and do not penalise.
This is a response to the qi of spring
And the Art of caring for life.

逆之則傷肝, 夏為實寒變, 奉長者少.

If you go against it you injure your liver.
In the summer the weather will stay wintry, and there is little to
    support any growth.

Li Zhongzi: The order of the four seasons is spring – birth; summer – growth;
autumn – closure; and winter – storage. To use these several rules is to
encapsulate the arts and ways of caring for the qi of life.

夏三月, 此為蕃秀.

During summer there are three moons,

This is a time for blooming and blossoming.

天地氣交, 萬物華實.
夜臥早起, 無厭于日,
使志勿怒, 使華英成秀, 使氣得泄, 若所愛在外.
此夏氣之應, 養長之道.

The qi of the skies and the earth can interpenetrate,

And all myriad creatures strengthen and flower.

Go to sleep at nightfall and rise in the dawn, do not be tired out
by the sun.

In such a way you enable your will to be freed from anger,

And help flower forth lushly into full blossom, and let it out and
go –

Just as if you loved all that lay beyond you.

This is a response to the qi of summer

And the Art of caring for growth.

逆之則傷心, 秋為痎瘧, 奉收者少, 冬至重病.

If you go against it you injure your heart.

In the autumn you suffer coughing and repeated fevers, and there
is little to support any closure.

Then winter arrives and heavy sickness.

秋三月, 此謂容平.

During the autumn there are three moons,

This is a time for sizing and settling.

天氣以急, 地氣以明.
早臥早起, 與雞俱興.
使志安寧, 以緩秋刑, 收斂神氣,
使秋氣平, 無外其志, 使肺氣清.
此秋氣之應, 養收之道也.

The heavenly qi is hastening,

The earthly qi is strengthening.

Go to bed early and rise up early,

Copying the behaviour of the cock.
In such a way you enable your will to stay peaceful and delay the
   penalty of the autumn.
Keep close and take in your mental strength
To enable the settling of the autumn.
Do not allow your thoughts to stray without,
To enable the lung qi to clear.
This is a response to the qi of the autumn,
And the Art of caring for closure.

逆之則傷肺, 冬為飧泄, 奉藏者少.
If you go against this you injure your lungs.
In the winter you suffer from diarrhoea and there is little to
   support any storage.

冬三月, 此為閉藏.
During winter there are three moons,
This is the time for storage and shutting up.

水冰地坼, 勿擾乎陽.
早臥晚起, 必待日光.
使志若伏若匿, 若有私意, 若已有得.
去寒就溫, 無泄皮膚, 使氣極奪.
此冬氣之應, 養藏之道也.
The streams freeze over and the soil cracks open,
Do not dare disturb the Yang.
Go to bed early and rise up late,
You must wait for a sight of the sun.
In such a way you enable your will to be subdued and hidden
   away –
As if you had secret thoughts,
As if your ideas were of what you had already attained.
Flee the cold weather and draw near the warmth,
Not letting the skin perspire at its surface.
Thus you enable the qi not to steal constantly away.
This is a response to the qi of winter,
And the Art of caring for storage.

逆之則傷腎, 春為痿厥, 奉生者少.

If you go against this you injure your kidneys.

In the spring there is wasting and withering, and little to support any life.

This section beginning with 'in springtime there are three moons' explains, in nuanced fashion, the responses of humankind to the passage of the year. There is a 'mutual interaction' 相应 *xiangying* or exchange between our internal organs – the five 'treasuries' 臟 *zang* or organ systems of traditional Chinese medicine (heart, lungs, kidneys, spleen and liver) – and nature. We have the rise and fall of Yin and Yang within us, echoing the world outside. The shifting sun and moon, arrival and departure of day and night, warmth and coolness of heated summer days and winter nights, these impinge on us all.

Playing on a theme of self-responsibility, the seasons reveal a rhythm. Their regularity is achieved through tolerating change. There is a marked mode to life, naturally stepped to the beat of Yin and Yang. Above there is the sky, with its moving constellations – below, the shifting seasons of the year. How can we sustain mental power and strength? Simply by watching nature. Observe the common pattern: birth and growth in spring and summer, closure and storage in autumn and winter. 'Birth and growth, closure and storage' 生長, 收藏 *shengzhang, shouzang* – these four characters depict the *yinyang* code for the world, as for all human society. Through them we learn an added dimension of care – understand the demands of the moment and adapt appropriately to the true but shifting connection with things. We know to care for birth, growth, closure and storage – and thus avoid harm.

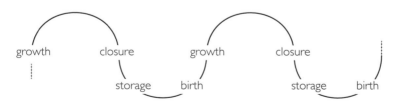

– summer – autumn – winter – spring – summer – autumn – winter – spring –

The Yin and Yang of birth and growth, closure and storage

RHYTHM OF LIFE

	three moons of spring	three moons of summer	three moons of autumn	three moons of winter
the natural world	the skies and the earth both give birth and all myriad creatures prosper	the skies and the earth can interpenetrate, and all myriad creatures strengthen and flower	the heavenly energies are hastening, the earthly strengthening	the streams freeze and the soil cracks open, do not dare disturb the Yang
its action	breaking out and bursting	blooming and blossoming	sizing and settling	storage and shutting up
sleep and wake	sleep at nightfall and rise at dawn, take large steps out in the courtyard, uncoil your hair and stretch out the body	go to sleep at nightfall and rise in the dawn, do not be tired out by the sun	go to bed early and rise up early, copying the behaviour of the cock	go to bed early and rise up late, you must wait for a sight of the sun
recipes for life	help bring forth life and do not slaughter, help donate and do not take away, help reward and do not penalise	help them to flower forth lushly into full blossom, and be let out and go – just as if you loved all that lay beyond you	keep close and take in your mental energies, do not allow your thoughts to stray without	as if you had secret thoughts, as if your ideas were of what you had already attained
the will and emotion	set the will on birth	enable your will to be freed from anger	enable your will to stay peaceful	enable your will to be subdued and hidden away
care path	caring for life	caring for growth	caring for closure	caring for storage
organ affect	if you go against this, you injure your liver	if you go against this, you injure your heart	if you go against this, you injure your lungs	if you go against this, you injure your kidneys
resultant	there is little to support any growth, and in summer the weather stays wintry	there is little to support any closure, and in the autumn coughing and repeated fevers, winter arrives and heavy sickness	there is little to support storage, and in the winter you suffer from diarrhoea	there is little to support any new life, in the spring there is wasting and withering

5. The Energy of the Yang Stored up

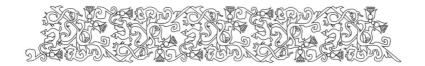

天氣清淨, 光明者也.
藏德不止, 故不下也.
天明則日月不明, 邪害空竅.

THE QI OF THE SKIES is clear and pure,
It is brilliant and shining!
It has a virtue stored up unceasing and inextinguishable.
But if the skies were to shine of themselves,
And the sun and moon not to shine,
The malign *xie* would enter in and harm would come to them
Through entering in through an opening.

陽氣者閉塞, 地氣者冒明, 雲霧不精, 則上應白露不下.

The Yang qi would block off,
The earthly qi be obscured.
Clouds and mists neither rise nor distil,
And then neither the clear dew descend.

交通不表, 萬物命故不施.

Then their interpenetration not externalised,
The life of the myriad creatures is not bestowed.

Wang Bing: The heavens store up virtue, as they wish to conceal their great light; if the great light was seen, so the small lights would perish.

Li Zhongzi: This is just speaking of the source of qi in the body. If its root is not stored up in the individual, it issues forth, exalted on the outside, and there is an opening in the light – and the malign *xie* runs in.

不施則名木多死, 惡氣不發, 風雨不節, 白露不下.

And if their life is not bestowed,

The many famed forests will fail.

Their polluted qi does not emerge,

Storms and rain-clouds arrive unchecked and the clear dew not
    descend.

則菀槁不榮, 賊風數至, 暴雨數起.

天地四時不相保, 與道相失, 則未央絕滅.

So then growth withers in the bud and none are able to prosper.

The thieving winds arrive endlessly and storms constantly arise.

The skies, the earth and four seasons

Offer each other no mutual support –

They lose track of each other,

And not even midway along their path any order collapses.

唯聖人從之, 故身無奇病, 萬物不失, 生氣不竭.

Only the Sages may comply with this,

Their bodies thus kept from obstinate disease.

Not one of the myriad creatures is neglected,

And their life force inexhaustible.

This extract delves further into the nature of the *yinyang*. Yang is the source of life – just as light and warmth bring growth in the spring. However, although all life comes from the Yang, it must also depend on the Yin – just as a man and woman are both needed to make a child.

The text says that 'if the skies were to shine of themselves and the sun and moon not to shine' they leave themselves open to attack. The heavens use the sun and moon to give light. But although the Yang is seen in the sun and moon, they have their rise and fall, their fullness and decline. It is only natural that the Yang has a need for rest. This is why the skies are able to 'store up virtue unceasing'. The Yang must never lose touch with the Yin – otherwise it would become brittle and break.

There is a natural purity residing in the humble heart, which is also Yang. Health relies on being not just strong but also kind, and listening to the other as well as to ourselves (Yang = self, Yin = other). We cannot just be strong and affirmative – it is important that we have a base and rhythm to our activity. Thus the *Yijing* states: 'the superior fellow first gets lost – then, later he gains a direction' (Hexagram 2, *Kun* – The Receptive). The interpenetration of Yin and Yang, like the mixing of qi and blood, allows the opportunity for survival, just as it enables any of us to find the balance and homeostasis of good health. If the Yang heavens were to attempt to shine of themselves, and be over-arrogant, the sun and moon would no longer shine but be eclipsed and all tangled up – as the malign *xie* creeps in.

We are told 'the famed forests would fail' and 'storms and rain-clouds arrive unchecked', showing a world in which Yin and Yang fight for power – where the Yang qi is ramped up and goes unbestowed. It is only through following the example of the Sages, by being both robust and gentle, that we can comply with the rhythm of nature – that is, competently handle both Yin and Yang, and thereby realise the Arts and ways of a good life.

6. The Practice of
Advancing the Yang

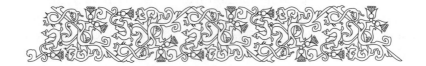

年四十, 而陰氣自半也, 起居衰矣.

WHEN YOU ARE FORTY YEARS OLD, the Yin qi itself
Makes up one half of you and your daily routine declines.

Li Zhongzi: Yin and Yang are the root origin of living and killing. Yang is the root of life, Yin is the foundation of death. When Yang prevails over Yin, you are strong; if Yin prevails over Yang, you decline. When Yin and Yang are half by half, signs of decline will be evident.

年五十, 體重, 耳目不聰明矣.

When you are fifty years old, the body grows heavier,
And your ears and eyes are not so sharp and clear.

Li Dongyuan: As you reach fifty or more, the qi which subdues you is greater and the qi which raises you up is lesser.

Zhang Jiebin: Yang commands life, Yin commands death. Yang commands growth, Yin commands dispersal. Yang commands rising, Yin commands falling. The Sages acted in accord with both.

Li Zhongzi: The Yang qi is lighter and tends to movement, the Yin qi is heavier and make it difficult to stretch out and be comfortable. At fifty the Yin qi is filling and hence the body becomes heavier.

年六十, 陰痿, 氣大衰, 九竅不利, 下虛上實, 涕泣俱出矣.

When you are sixty years old, the sexual force withers
And your breath and qi greatly subside.

The 'nine openings' do not work as effectively;
Weakened below and full above, you become incontinent.

Li Zhongzi: You weaken below as the lesser fire (kidney Yang) is weak. You fill above as the Yin rides on the Yang.

故曰: 知之則強, 不知則老, 故同出而名異耳.
智者察同, 愚者察異.
Therefore the saying:
Those who understand grow strong,
Those who misunderstand grow old.
These two come from a similar source,
And merely differ in name.
The wise discern the similarities,
The stupid discern the differences.

Li Zhongzi: Those wise penetrate the cause of Yin and Yang, and hence discern the similarities. Those stupid merely look at the outer appearances, stronger or weaker, and hence discern the differences.

愚者不足, 智者有餘, 有餘則耳目聰明, 身體輕強.
老者復壯, 壯者益治. 是以聖人為無為之事, 樂恬憺之能.
The stupid have insufficient, the wise have more than enough.
Having more than enough, their ears and eyes
Remain sharp and clear, their bodies light and strong.
Although they grow older, they remain vigorous;
And as they remain vigorous, they can further heal.
In this fashion the Sage conducts his business through the action
    of non-action,
And delights in his capacity for detachment and peace.

Li Zhongzi: As they remain vigorous, they can further heal – this is the idea behind 'giving up one's own ideas' and 'the growth of virtue' mentioned by Laozi.

Li Zhongzi: It is non-action which defines the self-made path. This is the 'non-action' of Laozi in which 'nothing is left undone'. It is the 'perfect delight' of Zhuangzi through which greatness is attained.

從欲快志於虛无之守.

故壽命无窮, 與天地終. 此聖人之治身也.

He follows his desires with a cheerful will, guarding the Void
within.

Hence his longevity and destiny are inexhaustible.

He ends his days along with the skies and the earth,

This is how the Sage heals his own body.

To 'end our days along with the skies and the earth' points to the
Taoist ecstasy, the blending of Yin and Yang, fluids and fire (our
metabolism), within our body. The whole of this *Suwen* chapter
explains the natural agencies of Yin and Yang, in life and decline.
The Yang, being warming and enlivening, is of direct importance
for health. The text encourages us to be watchful of the Yang at
middle age, linking it to a certain wisdom. Detachment and the
'action of non-action' 爲無爲 *wei wuwei* are discussed in *Laozi* 37.
The 'giving up of one's own ideas', which Li Zhongzi mentions,
comes from *Laozi* 59: 'In governing the people and serving heaven,
nothing is as good as forbearance, but forbearance is only the
habit of giving up one's own ideas, while giving up one's own ideas
brings about the growth of virtue. ' This practice was inherent
in the Taoist arts of 'inner alchemy' 內丹 *neidan*, as outlined in
the next section. Li Zhongzi quotes from the famous physician
Huato (140–208 CE) when he says, 'Yang is the root of life; Yin
the foundation of death. '

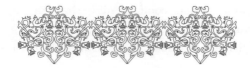

7. Taoist Yoga

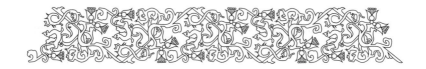

腎有久病者, 可以寅時面向南,
淨神不亂, 思閉氣不息七徧.

WHEN THE KIDNEYS HAVE BEEN ILL over a long period,
You must face south an hour before dawn.
Clear the mind, not allowing any unruly thoughts
And stop up the breath, seven times in all.

以引頸嚥氣順之, 如嚥氣甚硬物.
如此七徧後, 餌舌下津令無數.

Then stretch out the neck, gently swallowing the breath down –
Like swallowing a solid object.
After performing this practice seven times,
Take the saliva down, again and again, with the tongue.

Li Zhongzi: If the mind has no unruly thoughts, the heart will come close to
the Great Void – it becomes still and settled, and congealed into one. To stop
up the breath is to halt the passage of the breathing. As the breath reaches
its extreme point, very gently you push it on a little, without making a sound.
The breath is mother to the fluids, and the fluids the foundation of all life. Hard
work at this will extend your own life.

This section instructs us in four things: stilling the mind,
lengthening the breath, stretching the neck and swallowing
saliva. These practices are very old, their origins well before the
Han dynasty. Famous silk hangings and texts recovered from the
Mawangdui tombs, Hunan Province, suggest these skills went
back at least to the Warring States.

This text comes from one of the *Suwen*'s 'lost chapters'. It is not in the SWYS but is in the NJZY. They were lost before the Wang Bing compilation of 762 CE, and only their titles noted. Evidently they were replaced before Lin Yi's editing around 1050 CE. There is strong suspicion they were fabricated (or re-composed) and then inserted. This section advocates the common Taoist practice of lengthening the breath and swallowing saliva. The lungs are mother to the kidneys on the *wuxing* generative cycle. Thus the Yang breath (from the lungs) can nourish the Yin fluids (water of the kidneys). Li Zhongzi points out that 'the fluids are the foundation of all life'. He quotes from the inner alchemist Zhang Boduan: 'To swallow down saliva and take in breath are human activities, yet here is prescribed a medicine which can actually create life; however, if you have no true spark under your stove, it is like firing an empty pan!' This speaks of the inner development of the Adept. Have no 'true spark' means having no vitality. Li Zhongzi concludes: 'It feeds into a wondrous foundation while the qi feeds into a spirit. It is the kernel and "true spark". ' The *jing* 精 or 'spark' resides in the kidneys and gives us a fund for growth, reproduction and physical and mental development. This is why it is referred to as 'a wondrous foundation'.

8. The Sages Treated those Well, not those Sick

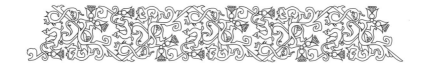

是故聖人不治已病, 治未病, 不治已亂, 治未亂, 此之謂也.
夫病已成而後藥之, 亂已成而後治之,
譬猶渴而穿井, 鬪而鑄錐, 不亦晚乎.

AND THE SAGES DID NOT treat those already sick,
They treated them before they were sick.
In government they did not deal with a catastrophe after it had
    arrived,
They dealt with it before it had happened.
This is a commonly known fact.

Therefore, when sickness has begun to take hold and you
    medicate,
Or when a catastrophe has taken hold and you attempt to govern,
It is like being thirsty and looking to dig a well,
Or casting weapons on the way into battle.
This is just too late!

Chinese medicine is traditionally seen as preventative. It excels in
the use of tonics to maintain a tenuous hold on health. There is
the old adage that you paid your Chinese doctor when you were
well – and stopped paying when you fell sick. What use is it to
wait until becoming thirsty before you dig a well? Or to look for
weapons on the way into battle? The metaphor is blunt.

9. The Character of the Malign *Xie* or Thief-Wind

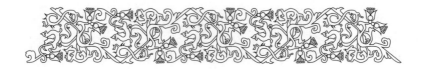

風從南方來, 名曰大弱風. 風從西南方來, 名曰謀風.
風從西方來, 名曰 剛風. 風從西北方來, 名曰折風.
風從北方來, 名曰大剛風. 風從東北方來, 名曰凶風.
風從東方來, 名曰嬰兀風. 風從東南方來, 名曰弱風.

AS THE WIND COMES FROM A SOUTHERLY
   DIRECTION,
The world knows it as the Greatly Enfeebling Wind.
As the wind comes from a south-westerly direction,
The world knows it as the Plotting Wind.
As the wind comes from a westerly direction,
The world knows it as the Stiffening Wind.
As the wind comes from a north-westerly direction,
The world knows it as the Cutting Wind.
As the wind comes from a northern direction,
The world knows it as the Greatly Stiffening Wind.
As the wind comes from a north-easterly direction,
The world knows it as the Malicious Wind.
As the wind comes from an easterly direction,
The world knows it as the Entangling Wind.
As the wind comes from a south-easterly direction,
The world knows it as the Enfeebling Wind.

Zhang Jiebin: The whole of this passage describes how when we are weakened and caught by the wind, it invades and creates a sickness within.

This last extract is from *Lingshu* 77, the companion volume to the *Suwen*. It describes the eight directions of the compass, and the characters of their malign *xie* winds. I have omitted the paragraphs attached to each wind describing the ailments caused. During recent excavations a jade disc has been found in a grave at Lingjiatan, Anhui, dated to c. 3000 BCE. It probably depicts cosmological thinking – and in its depiction of the four (or eight) directions (and centre) it shows the beginnings of an appreciation of 'place'. It is the earliest reference to a graphical representation of the eight directions, later linked to the 'eight trigrams', that I have found.

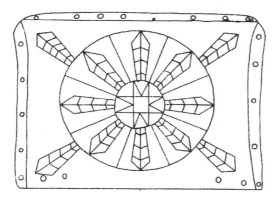

Early depiction of the eight directions

When the climate is unstable or out of true, it reveals an imbalance which can 'invade' our bodies. In a very real sense, the task of keeping well lies in paying attention to the detail: light and dark, warmth and cold and seasonal change – a clear awareness, lived out in a fluctuating world. In other words, regulate your sleep and activity, wear appropriate clothing, take time out occasionally, and watch what you eat. Xue Shengbai sums up this chapter:

> In all the myriad scrolls of the *Suwen* and *Lingshu*, there is not one single character which is not concerned with the secret of honouring life. These extracts are not put together by chance but concern the business of 'guarding the One'. They are not

venerating any other aspect but the 'three strangers' – the Way, the Yin and Yang. Generally speaking, you will find that the most important task is to advance your years along with the age-old methods of honouring life. View the pathway of the heavens and you may grasp their cycle, this is everything. But an understanding not founded on 'humility and a deep sense of peace' leads directly to the malign arts. If you do not return to 'easy and simple' methods you are only exploring byways. In all truth if you search out the essence, you need no other books – not even the five thousand-word *Tao-te Ching*, nor the myriad writings of the alchemists!

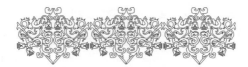

Questions for Review of Chapter I
* Indicates a more challenging question

1. What is the first lesson the Yellow Emperor is given by his counsellor Qi Bo concerning moderation, the Yin and Yang?

2. How does illness arrive? How are illness and weakness combined?

3. What were the four types of 'ancient Sages', the ideal people of old? Describe and illustrate their qualities.

4. Make an extensive discussion on Zhang Jiebin's statement, 'one's heart is one's own, unmoved'. *

5. In a few words sum up the 'conservative' attitude of the 'Ancients'. Draw, if you wish, on your own experience. Can you think why the ancient Chinese were so concerned with the preservation of life?

6. Describe in a few lines how the 'rhythm of the seasons' applies to your own life. It may help if you first list the separate qualities of caring for 'life, growth, closure and storage'.

7. How does 'life, growth, closure and storage' apply to the world at present?

8. Why does the Yang need to be 'stored up'? What has this to do with the purity of the heart?*

9. What are we advocated to do to 'advance the Yang'? Why then do we also foster the Yin fluids of the kidney (as in Taoist Yoga)?

10. Expand on the characters of the winds and climates from the 'eight directions'.

Characters in Chapter I

Yin, Yang 陰陽 *yinyang*

Five Elements 五行 *wuxing*

ancient Sages 古聖 *gusheng*

weak, empty condition 虛 *xu*

malign, perverse or pathogenic factor 邪 *xie*

real qi 真氣 *zhen qi*

mental strength, mind 精神 *jingshen*

people of real substance 真人 *zhen ren*

Adepts 至人 *zhi ren*

Sages 聖人 *sheng ren*

the Wise ones 賢人 *xian ren*

mutual interaction, exchange (between internal organs and nature, and so on) 相应 *xiangying*

birth and growth, closure and storage 生長, 收藏 *shengzhang, shouzang*

action of non-action 爲無爲 *wei wuwei*

inner alchemy 內丹 *neidan*

spark, or vitality (resides in the kidneys) 精 *jing*

II

Yin and Yang

If you scrutinise the intricacies of Yin and Yang, and regulate the empty and full, the root of sickness lies in the palm of your hand and the blessed medical scrolls find their place in your heart.

Key Ideas

1. *Yin and Yang, the Way of the Skies and Earth*
   Yin and Yang, a clear mind, seeking the root, accumulation, transformation, completion, heat and cold, clear and turbid

2. *Yin and Yang, Water, Fire, Qi and Flavours*
   the *yinyang* in the body, clear and turbid, skin, *zangfu* organs, limbs, qi, *jing*, flavours, thick and thin, the development of heat, a vigorous fire, a lesser fire, injury differentiation

3. *Left and Right as different as North and South*
   the body, reflecting the skies and earth, wind, rain

4. *Yin and Yang in the Skies and Man*
   the *yinyang*, the day and night, the body, the *zangfu*

5. *The Crucial Importance of the Yang Needing Rest*
   the Yang, skies and sun, the propriety of Yin and Yang, dense-packed, mental equilibrium

Some questions for review can be found at the end of this chapter.

1. Yin and Yang, the Way of the Skies and Earth

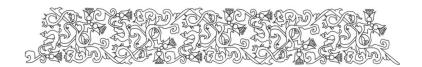

陰陽者天地之道也, 萬物之綱紀也, 變化之父母,
生殺之本始, 神明之府也. 治病必求於本.

YIN AND YANG FORM THE WAY of the skies and earth.
They make up the rules and patterns for the myriad creatures.
They are the father and mother
Of all change and transformation,
The root origin of living and killing,
They are the treasury of a clear mind.
In treating sickness you must seek for the root.

Zhang Zhicong: The root means the root of Yin and Yang. The *zangfu*, qi and blood, inner and outer, upper and lower divisions of man all find their root in Yin and Yang. While without we are assailed by the wind, cold, summer warmth and damp, the four seasons and *wuxing* again derive totally from the two qi of Yin and Yang. Whether concerned with treating disease through herbs or diet, or applying the needle, whether you are examining colour and pulse or making a medical case from their social standing, it all lies in the province of Yin and Yang. Thus the text says, 'to treat sickness, you must seek for the root'.

Li Zhongzi: Unfathomable in change and transformation, this is the meaning of 'mind'; materiality flowing into form, this is the meaning of 'clear'. A treasury signifies a flowing into form, change and transformation. Everything can be deduced from this.

Li Zhongzi: All humankind is beset by sickness. Although it has no single cause, sickness either belongs to the category of the weak (*xu*) or strong (*shi*), cold or heat, the qi or blood, to the *zang* or *fu*, and all are contained in the Yin and

Yang. For that reason, although our understanding of sickness alters constantly,
Yin and Yang remain the root.

故積陽為天, 積陰為地. 陰靜陽燥, 陽生陰長, 陽殺陰藏.

This being so an accumulation of Yang forms the skies
While an accumulation of the Yin forms the earth.
The Yin is still and the Yang impetuous,
The Yang gives birth and the Yin matures.
The Yang to destroy, the Yin to conceal.

Li Zhongzi: The Yin itself never acts singly – it follows the Yang then acts. Just
as the 'shutting away and storage' of the cold winter follows on entirely from
the destruction wrought by the autumn storms and frosts. So it says in the text:
'The Yang to destroy, the Yin to conceal. '

陽化氣, 陰成形.

The Yang provides a transforming qi,
The Yin completes the form.

Li Zhongzi: Yang has no form, so it makes up the transforming qi. Yin has
substance, so it completes the forms of things.

寒極生熱, 熱極生寒.

Extreme cold generates heat,
Extreme heat generates cold.

Li Zhongzi: The extreme cold of winter brings about the warmth of spring and
summer. The extreme heat of summer brings about the cold of autumn and
winter.

寒氣生濁, 熱氣生清.

Cold qi creates turbidity,
Heated qi creates clarity.

Li Zhongzi: Cold belongs to the Yin, so it creates turbidity. Heat belongs to the
Yang, so it creates clarity.

清氣在下, 則生飧泄, 濁氣在上, 則生膹脹.

While a clear qi is found below,
It creates diarrhoea with undigested food.

When a turbid qi is found above,
It creates staring eyes and a distending headache.

Li Zhongzi: The clear Yang should ascend. As it sinks below, it cannot ascend
and food becomes undigested. The turbid Yin should descend. As it reverses
above, it can no longer descend. It turns into staring eyes and a distending
headache. The chest and diaphragm feel swollen and full.

There is one grand principle common to all threads of Chinese
medicine – the principle of Yin and Yang (陰陽 *yinyang*). Along
with the idea of the Tao (or 'Way') and the qi, Yin and Yang give
us an explanation for how the world works. The *yinyang* signifies
a complementary but shifting balance between contraries – as it
forms 'the Way of the skies and earth'. The phenomenon of the
circling skies is the picture of change – and yet this change itself
is also constant. In addition, within the body, Yin and Yang come
together and fall apart, rise and fall – as in the moving blood (Yin)
and qi (Yang) in the *zang* 臟, or solid, and *fu* 腑, more hollow,
organs – and yet their principle remains the same. The opening
line above, 'Yin and Yang form the Way of the skies and earth',
begins *Suwen* 5, entitled 'On the Resonant Phenomena of Yin and
Yang'. This chapter explains that Yin and Yang are the 'treasury of
a clear mind' – and also that in order to treat sickness, you 'must
seek for the root' 必求於本 *biqiu yuben*, the root in the Yin and
Yang.

Critically, the Han scholars who assembled the *Suwen*
developed *yinyang* and *wuxing* thinking to categorise and
synthesise all data. Yin and Yang formed the backbone on which
could be hung traditional Chinese science. The exigencies of
the *yinyang* grew into an intricate but vastly flexible system,
enabling the pigeonholing of experience – making best use of a
searching intellect. The *yinyang* tool allows work on ourselves at
the same time as it helps us observe the universe. This is truly
an 'investigation of things' or *gewu* (see earlier). The implication
is that to learn medicine correctly, we must be self-reflective. As
we gain a clearer view of the world, so also, concurrently, we
gain insight into ourselves. This is the feat of Chinese traditional

medicine – that it compounds both a Confucian self-scrutiny and a Taoist fascination with how life comes about. Yin and Yang *by nature* imply reflective practice. Their dialogue implies work done towards 'a clear mind' 神明 *shenming*. *Shenming* has many translations, but it is obvious from Li Zhongzi's commentary that in this context it means clear thinking.

THE *YINYANG*

the Way	of the skies and earth
the rules and patterns	for the myriad creatures
the father and mother	of all change and transformation
the root origin	of living and killing
the treasury	of a clear mind

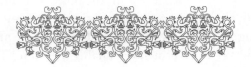

2. Yin and Yang, Water, Fire, Qi and Flavours

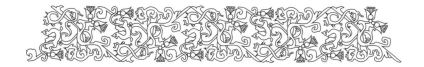

清陽為天, 濁陰為地, 地氣上為雲, 天氣下為雨.

THE CLEAR YANG FORMS THE SKIES,
The turbid Yin represents the earth.
The earthly qi rises above to form the clouds,
The qi of the skies descends as rain.

Li Zhongzi: The skies and earth are spoken of in terms of 'clouds and rain'; the human body is spoken of in terms of *jing* and qi. The human body is as one single small universe. Now do you understand?

故清陽出上竅, 濁陰出下竅, 清陽發腠理, 濁陰走五臟.
清陽實四肢, 濁陰歸六腑.

The clear Yang comes out from the upper openings,
The turbid Yin comes out from the lower openings.
The clear Yang develops into the texture of the skin,
While the turbid Yin runs back to the five *zang*.
The clear Yang gives substance to the four limbs,
While the turbid Yin returns to the six *fu*.

Li Zhongzi: The Yang entirely establishes without, the Yin entirely establishes within.

水為陰, 火為陽.
陽為氣, 陰為味, 味歸形, 形歸氣.

Water is Yin; fire is Yang.
The Yang forms the qi,

The Yin forms the tastes.
The tastes go back to the physical body,
So the body goes back to the qi.

Li Zhongzi: Water seeps below and is cooling, thus Yin. Fire blazes above and is heating, thus Yang. What blazes above is at the point of sinking below and what is seeping below is at the point of rising above. This is the meaning of water and fire mixing together and triumphing in the body. The kidneys deal with water and within this water are born our qi, namely the 'true fire'. The heart deals with fire and within this fire is born a fluid, namely the 'true waters'. Yang in Yin and Yin in Yang. Waters and fires, Yin and Yang both linked in the body. This you must understand.

Li Zhongzi: The tastes 'go back to the physical body' because food entering the mouth creates blood and builds up the physical form. The body 'goes back to the qi' because blood is entirely dependent on qi. As the qi is strong it can, of itself, create blood. If the qi is injured, the blood as a consequence will decline.

氣歸精, 精歸化.
The qi goes back to the *jing*;
The *jing* goes back to the transformations.

Zhang Jiebin: The qi here is the 'true qi' 真氣 *zhenqi*, that which we receive at birth. It combines together with the qi from food to fill up the body. The human body is composed of *jing* and qi. From the qi we gain transformation. Thus the qi goes back to the *jing*.

Li Zhongzi: The qi here is the 'source qi' 元氣 *yuanqi* we are born with. It combines with the acquired qi we get from food to fill up the body…the *jing* is the 'true lead of Kan's palace', the single line in the trigram Water, and the first and foremost evidence of our oneness with nature. As this *jing* is bestowed upon us, so it is able to effect all transformations of life. This is the root cause of all life.

精食氣, 形食味.
The *jing* feeds off the qi,
The physical body feeds off the tastes.

Li Zhongzi: The qi acts as mother to the *jing*. The tastes we eat form the foundation for the body. So the body feeds off them, just as a child feeds off its mother's milk.

化生精, 氣生形.

The transformations are created from *jing*.

So qi creates the physical body.

味傷形, 氣傷精.

The tastes may injure the body,

The qi may injure the *jing*.

Li Zhongzi: The tastes fundamentally 'go back to the physical body'. If perhaps the tastes are not checked, instead they injure the body. The qi fundamentally 'goes back to the *jing*'. If perhaps the qi is not harmonised, instead it injures the *jing*.

精化為氣, 氣傷於味.

The *jing* transforms into qi,

The qi is injured by the tastes.

Li Zhongzi: The qi fundamentally 'goes back to the *jing*' – so it acts as mother to the *jing*. Here it says 'the *jing* transforms into qi', meaning that *jing* may also create qi. For instance, if you do not show a great fondness for sexual activity it means your qi may find a way to flourish. Water and fire are linked at root. This is the significance of the above text where it mentions the image of 'the skies and the earth, clouds and rain'.

陰味出下竅, 陽氣出上竅.

The Yin tastes come out from the lower openings,

The Yang qi comes out from the upper openings.

味厚者為陰, 薄為陰之陽. 氣厚者為陽, 薄為陽之陰.
味厚則泄, 薄則通. 氣薄則發泄, 厚則發熱.

Tastes which thicken up are more Yin,

Those which thin out are more Yang than Yin.

Qi which thickens up is more Yang,

That which thins out is more Yin than Yang.

Tastes which thicken up are passed out below,

As they thin out they permeate the whole body.

Qi which thins out is also eliminated.

If it thickens up it develops as heat.

Li Zhongzi: Qi which thins out can be eliminated outside; qi which thickens up can develop into heat.

壯火之氣衰, 少火之氣壯, 壯火食氣, 氣食少火,
壯火散氣, 少火生氣.

In a vigorous fire the qi is weakened,
In a lesser fire the qi is strengthened.
A vigorous fire consumes the qi,
The qi consumes a lesser fire.
A vigorous fire scatters the qi,
While a lesser fire generates qi.

Li Zhongzi: Fire means Yang qi…if things are to be born, they must be rooted in the Yang. But only the fire of a peaceful Yang can give birth to things. A blazing fire will harm them. Therefore if the fire is too strong, the qi instead declines; if the fire is peaceful, the qi strengthens. A vigorous fire scatters the qi…so it 'consumes the qi'; a lesser fire generates qi…so the 'qi consumes a lesser fire'.

Li Zhongzi: Therefore if the fire is too strong, instead the qi declines; if the fire is peacefully balanced, the qi is strengthened.

陰勝則陽病, 陽勝則陰病, 陽勝則熱, 陰勝則寒.
重寒則熱, 重熱則寒.

As Yin predominates, so Yang is sick,
As Yang predominates, so Yin is sick.
As Yang predominates there is heat,
As Yin predominates there is cold.
Severe cold generates heat,
Severe heat generates cold.

Li Zhongzi: As Yin and Yang intermingle, so they arrive at the norm. An imbalance in either precipitates sickness. In the interchange of Yin and Yang, water at its extreme resembles fire, while fire at its extreme resembles water. When Yang is full it cuts out Yin, and when Yin is full it cuts out Yang. So then there appear the symptoms of real cold within and false heat outside, or real heat within and false cold outside. If you do not discern how they have interchanged, but recklessly hand over the prescription, it is like deepening the water or building up the fire! Although you may be wise in learning, you cannot save them from disaster.

寒傷形, 熱傷氣.

Coldness injures the body,

Heat injures the qi.

Li Zhongzi: Coldness is Yin and the body is also Yin…heat is Yang and the qi is also Yang.

氣傷痛, 形傷腫,

If the qi is injured, there is pain,

If the body is injured, it creates swelling.

Li Zhongzi: The qi excels at passing through. If it is injured it may become blocked and cannot pass through, causing pain.

故先痛而後腫者氣傷形也,

先腫而後痛者形傷氣也.

Thus if first pain and later swelling,

It is the qi injuring the body,

If first swelling and later pain,

It is the body injuring the qi.

喜怒傷氣, 寒暑傷形.

Pleasure and anger injure the qi,

Cold and summer heat injure the body.

The Yang forms the skies above, while the Yin consolidates the earth beneath. In the body, they appear as qi 氣 and *jing* 精. This is the basic sense of the atmosphere in our planet and life in our bodies. Though it is true the clear Yang forms the skies, according to the principle of the *yinyang*, where there is Yang, Yin cannot be far behind. Water is Yin, so we have rain and clouds. This thinking is further developed. For instance, in the body (the small 'heaven and earth') the turbid Yin 'comes out from the lower openings' through our bowels and bladder, while the clear Yang rises to the head and brightens the face and senses, to form our perception of the world.

Yin, being thicker, forms into tastes and food. But the Yang, being synonymous with qi, moves to transform food into blood, and so blood (Yin) and qi (Yang) circulate around together. In addition, the qi 'goes back to the *jing*'. They have their ultimate source in the kidneys. *Jing* is stored in the kidneys – and has much to do with fertility and development. The loins are the powerhouse of the body.

In brief, the tastes we eat 'go back to the physical body' just as food creates our physique, and the body 'goes back to the qi' just as the Yin blood is entirely dependent on the Yang qi. In addition, this qi 'goes back to the *jing*' just as qi depends for its power on *jing* – and the *jing* 'goes back to the transformations', just as it is responsible for all life. Yet in reciprocal fashion, the *jing* also 'feeds off the qi', as both qi and *jing* are bound together. The body 'feeds off the tastes' just as it depends on food for its survival. Last, the transformations of life are 'created from *jing*', just as all life comes from the central line of Kan ☵ (a symbol for the kidney Yang); and qi 'creates the physical body' just as it is able to carry into material form the potentiality of *jing*.

In the next few sections, this tortuous thinking is condensed further. Fundamentally, it reiterates the nature of the Yang. A *vigorous* Yang (qi or fire) can only decline – it is a *lesser* Yang which has the chance of growth and getting stronger. This is *yinyang* thinking. Within the kidneys, the real fire warms up the water; this is what keeps us warm and alive. Within the heart, the real water cools the fire; this is what keeps us 'in a cool temper'. This is how we achieve balance – in physiological terms: it describes the promotion of the *yinyang* homeostasis. Be watchful of the Yang, for it is a general truth in therapy that gentle encouragement can work better than enforced change – it can also be more invigorating! The qi 'consumes a lesser fire' because it literally 'feeds on', that is, develops from, a lesser fire.

Li Zhongzi makes the same point: 'If the fire is too strong, instead the qi declines; if the fire is peacefully balanced, the qi is strengthened. ' He goes on:

> The Yang qi means those warm and comfortable energies felt in the human body. If these ever terminate, the body will cool

down and life will come to an end. The *Neijing* repeatedly states this one simple truth. It intends mankind to become skilful at tending to the fire. Only a lesser fire becomes strong – a vigorous fire will decline. You must especially be skilful at regulating the flame and its heat.

Both Li Zhongzi and Zhang Jiebin see 'fire' and the Yang qi of the body as synonymous. They believe a lesser fire strengthens the body, reflecting the 'warming and tonifying' school of the Ming herbalists. It is their contention that a vigorous fire must be short-lived – whilst a gentle fire has a chance to grow. Li Zhongzi takes our natural birthright, or 'real fire' 真火 *zhen huo*, as the very stuff of our physiology. 'Real' 真 *zhen* here means 'original, untarnished, recovered'. These ideas were made much of by writers on *neidan* 內丹 or 'internal alchemy'.

A VIGOROUS FIRE, A LESSER FIRE

a vigorous fire	the qi is weakened
a lesser fire	the qi is strengthened
a vigorous fire	consumes the qi
the qi energy	consumes a lesser fire
a vigorous fire	scatters the qi
a lesser fire	generates the qi

3. Left and Right as different as North and South

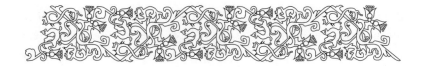

天不足西北, 故西北方陰也, 而人右耳目不如左明也.
地不滿東南, 故東南方陽也, 而人左手足不如右強也.
陽之汗以天地之雨名之, 陽之氣以天地之疾風名之.

THE SKIES ARE INSUFFICIENT to the north and west,
So the north-westerly regions are Yin –
Furthermore man's right ear and eye are not as sharp as his left.
The earth is incomplete to the south and east,
So the south-easterly regions are Yang –
Furthermore man's left hand is not as strong as his right.
The Yang sweat is named after the falling rain of the skies and
    earth.
The Yang qi is named after the swift wind of the skies and earth.

Li Zhongzi: The skies are Yang, and the north and west is Yin. Thus the skies are insufficient to the north and west. The earth is Yin, and the south and east are Yang. Thus the earth is incomplete to the south and east.

The skies are Yang and support the sun, also Yang. The sun rises in the east and travels across to the south. But because of the tilt of the ecliptic, the skies appear as 'insufficient to the north and west', as if they show a lack of Yang vigour. It is similar on the earth, where 'the south-easterly regions are Yang; that is, warmer. In other words, the contrasting characters of Yin and Yang are played out in the natural scheme of the world. As in the world, so in the body. In addition, by modelling the body on the natural world, the Yang sweat can be seen as 'falling rain' – while the qi emerges as the 'swift wind of the skies and earth'. The whole is analogy.

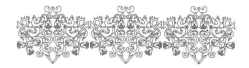

4. Yin and Yang in the Skies and Man

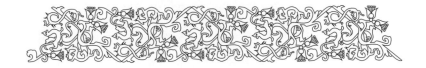

平旦至日中, 天之陽, 陽中之陽也, 日中至黃昏, 天之陽, 陽中之陰也.
日中至黃昏, 天之陽, 陽中之陰也, 合夜至雞鳴, 天之陰, 陰中之陰也.
雞鳴至平旦, 天之陰, 陰中之陽也.

DAWN UNTIL MIDDAY is the Yang of the skies:
The Yang within the Yang.
Midday until dusk is the Yang of the skies:
The Yin within the Yang.
Nightfall until cockcrow is the Yin of the skies:
The Yin within the Yin.
Cockcrow until dawn is the Yin of the skies:
The Yang within the Yin.

夫言人之陰陽, 則外為陽, 內為陰.
言人身之陰陽, 則背為陽, 腹為陰.
言人身之臟腑中陰陽, 則臟者為陰, 腑者為陽.
肝心脾肺腎五臟皆為陰, 膽胃大腸小腸膀胱三焦六腑皆為陽.

When speaking of Yin and Yang in man,
The outside is Yang and the inside is Yin.
When speaking of Yin and Yang in the body,
The back is Yang and the belly Yin.
When speaking of Yin and Yang within the *zangfu* of the body,
The *zang* are Yin and the *fu* are Yang.

The five *zang* – the liver, heart, spleen, lungs and kidneys – are all
   Yin;
The six *fu* – the gall, stomach, large intestines,
The small intestines, bladder and *sanjiao* –
They are all Yang.

故背為陽, 陽中之陽心也, 背為陽, 陽中之陰肺也.
腹為陰, 陰中之陰腎也, 腹為陰, 陰中之陽肝也.
腹為陰, 陰中之至陰脾也.

Therefore the back is Yang,
And the Yang within the Yang is the heart.
The back is Yang, and the Yin within the Yang are the lungs.
The belly is Yin, and the Yin within the Yin are the kidneys.
The belly is Yin, and the Yang within the Yin is the liver.
The belly is Yin, and the most Yin within the Yin is the spleen.

This section illustrates the proper use of the *yinyang* in timing
night and day. When the sun is up, the time is Yang; 'nightfall
until cockcrow' is the Yin (quiet) of the night. *Yinyang* thinking
also permeates the categorisation of the organs. The *zang* organs
are Yin (they store up, like a treasury), while the *fu* are Yang (they
move through). However, within these categories, the *yinyang* is
further at work: so the heart may be Yang (above) and the kidneys
Yin (below). This thinking is self-reflective and creative. When all
is flux during the consultation and treatment, we must be true
to the situation at hand – and clearly identify Yin and Yang in
our minds, accordingly. This shows the need to take great care
in practice.

YINYANG IN THE HEAVENS

dawn until midday	Yang of the skies	Yang within the Yang
midday until dusk	Yang of the skies	Yin within the Yang
nightfall until cockcrow	Yin of the skies	Yin within the Yin
cockcrow until dawn	Yin of the skies	Yang within the Yin

YINYANG IN THE HUMAN BODY

in man	outside is Yang	inside is Yin
in the body	back is Yang	belly is Yin
in the zangfu	the *fu* are Yang	the *zang* are Yin

5. The Crucial Importance of the Yang Needing Rest

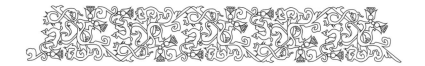

陽氣者, 若天與日, 失其所, 則折壽而不彰. 故天運當以日光明.

THE YANG QI IS LIKE UNTO the skies and the sun.

If it loses position, the length of our life is broken and we fail in
  influence.

Likewise the passage of the skies is matched by the sun, brilliant
  and shining.

凡陰陽之要, 陽密乃固, 兩者不和, 若春無秋若冬無夏.

Very generally the crucial nature of Yin and Yang

Means that if the Yang is dense-packed, our lives are solid.

If Yin and Yang are not peaceful together

It is like spring without autumn, or winter without summer.

因而和之, 是謂聖度.

Accordingly, if you bring them together,

You create what is known as 'Sagely moderation'.

故陽強不能密, 陰氣乃絕. 陰平陽秘, 精神乃治.

So if the Yang acts violently it cannot become dense-packed,

And the Yin qi comes to an end.

While if the Yin is balanced you may keep a tight hold on the
  Yang,

And the mind will find some peace.

Li Zhongzi: The Yin blood settled and still within, the Yang qi held and dense-packed without. If the Yin can nourish the *jing*, the Yang can nourish the mind. The *jing* once sufficient, your mind is your own – and life may be called peaceful.

Human life is entirely dependent on the proper maintenance of the Yang qi. Therefore it is critical that there is a rhythm to the Yang – there has to be a down-time. It is crucial that the Yang has a period when it is 'stored up', just as in the winter-time, and does not run on to become overbearing. Where Yang takes the lead, Yin will follow: this is a truth in all nature. Following Li Zhongzi, I omit several lines after the phrase 'brilliant and shining'. Li Zhongzi comments:

Yin on command, guarding within; Yang on command, shielding without. The Yang dense-packed is outside, so the malign *xie* can no longer invade; while the Yin is within, with a solid hold. When they are not at peace, it creates partiality. Partiality towards Yang is like spring without autumn; partiality towards Yin is like winter without summer. To bring both into harmony is to disperse excess and reinforce insufficiency. To enable no partiality or prominence is the rule of 'Sagely moderation'.

For the Chinese mind, nature and humankind are inextricably linked. Greatness means to accord with the natural movement of the skies and the year, to align ourselves with the sun and moon, echoing the rhythm of the seasons. This is to cultivate a 'Sagely moderation', as the Yang qi, being active, can easily expire if it loses touch with its Yin partner. The Yang needs to be 'dense-packed' outside. Yin means sleep and settling, and if the Yang is dense-packed, then the Yin can rest and be contained and protected. As Yin 'is balanced', you keep a tight hold on the Yang. In this fashion, 'your mind is your own and life may be called peaceful'. As the text says, 'if the Yin is balanced you may keep a tight hold on the Yang, and the mind will find some peace'. These lines illustrate the ultimate principle of *yinyang*, awake and asleep.

Li Zhongzi adds the implication that then the malign *xie* can no longer invade. Xue Shengbai comments:

> The medical classics are so many they would fill a house to its rafters! But there is nothing in them beyond Yin and Yang. Truly, the *zang* and the *fu*, belly and back, above and below; outer and inner body; left, right, 'foot', 'inch', floating, sinking, tardy and rapid pulses; the seasonal order of spring, summer, autumn and winter; the yearly shifting of the southern and northern parts of the sky – throughout all of these – if you scrutinise the intricacies of Yin and Yang, and regulate the empty and full, then the root of sickness will lie in the palm of your hand and the blessings of the medical scrolls be placed in your heart. It cannot be put plainer than this. I have omitted nothing. It is a thing so simple, and yet dependable on!

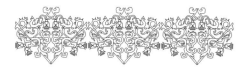

Questions for Review of Chapter II
* Indicates a more challenging question

1. First describe *at least* six characteristics of Yin and Yang. Then explain, briefly, how their modalities work within the human body.

2. How does Yin turbidity create disease?*

3. Expand on how the clear Yang and turbid Yin act in the body.

4. Describe *in detail* how water, fire, qi, *jing* and tastes (foodstuffs) all interact within the physical body. Be sure to explain how 'tastes' and energies can cause injury and illness. *

5. How did the Chinese explain the fact that one side of the body is stronger than the other?

6. How do Yin and Yang work in (a) the skies, (b) humans and (c) the *zangfu* organs?

Characters in Chapter II

Yin and Yang 陰陽 *yinyang*

solid organs 臟 *zang*

more hollow organs 腑 *fu*

you must seek for the root 必求於本 *biqiu yuben*

a clear mind, spiritual light (many translations) 神明 *shenming*

true qi 真氣 *zhenqi*

source qi 元氣 *yuanqi*

qi 氣 *qi*

jing 精 *jing*

real fire 真火 *zhen huo*

internal alchemy 內丹 *neidan*

III

Examining the Colour

Gazing at the facial colour comes first. Never by relying
solely on the pulse is it possible to effect treatment.

Key Ideas

1. *Purity, Brightness, Colour and Complexion*
   the qi in the face and eyes, purity and brightness, flowering
   and decline

2. *The Bright-lit Hall, the Physiognomy of Face*
   a detailed map, correspondences between face and *zangfu*,
   the 'glistening', colour, movement and character, pain, heat
   and cold, wind, *bi* immobility, weakness, fatality, puffiness,
   draining, drying out, breaking up, gathering

3. *The Basis of Health in the Face*
   the ubiquity of the soil (yellow)

Some questions for review can be found at the end of this chapter.

1. Purity, Brightness, Colour and Complexion

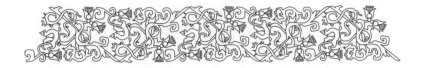

夫精明五色者, 氣之華也.

PURITY AND BRIGHTNESS and the 'five colours' reveal the flowering of the qi.

Wu Kun: Purity and brightness are shown in the eyes; the colours reveal themselves in the face. Both show if there is splendour and life in the qi.

赤欲如帛裹朱, 不欲如赭, 白欲如鵝羽, 不欲如鹽,
青欲如蒼璧之澤, 不欲如藍, 黃欲如羅裹雄黃, 不欲如黃土,
黑欲如重漆色, 不欲如地蒼.

Red must be like the colour of a scarlet silken wrapping, not reddish brown earth;

White must be like the colour of a white goose's wing, not ashen rock-salt;

Blue-green must be shining like a green jade emblem of rank, not like dark blue indigo;

Yellow must be the colour of bright yellow gauze, not like soil from the Yellow River;

Black must be the colour of a double layer of lacquer, not dullish grey earth.

五色精微象見矣, 其壽不久也.

If the image of a deteriorating purity in the five colours is seen, life will not last long.

Li Zhongzi: What is desirable in the 'five colours' is quite simply that they should be glistening – what is unwanted is that they deteriorate until they look withered and dried out.

夫精明者, 所以視萬物, 別白黑, 審短長.
以長為短, 以白為黑, 如是則精衰矣.
The term 'purity and brightness' above
Determines the method of observation:
Separate out the colour, deciding on its size and spread.
If there is some disclarity, or a mix in the spread, its purity is
    surely in decline.

Li Zhongzi: The purest qi of the *zangfu* rises upwards into the eyes and manifests as a shining and brilliant light. Thus the mention of a 'purity and brightness'. If this pure qi cannot ascend and rise, things are turned upside down in the body. How could there be anything left to support life?

Wu Kun: The image of 'a deteriorating purity seen' refers to a deterioration in the qi of the true source *jing*. Its energies transform, creating the shape of the colours revealed flowering outside. If they alter, they are not being bred within the *zang*. This shows the true qi is being shed. Therefore life will not last long.

This extract provides us with a view of the qi and blood in the body, and how they create the colour and complexion shown in the face. We may judge the health of the internal organs from the tenor, distribution and movement of colours on the face. In health they look moist and 'glistening' 潤澤 *runze*; in sickness they appear withered or dried up, implying a deterioration within. This text, along with the following, is the most ancient in the tradition of facial diagnosis. The lines above come from the *Suwen*; the following are from the *Lingshu*.

FLOWERING OF THE QI

complexion	must be like	must not be like
red	scarlet silken wrapping	reddish-brown earth
white	a white goose's wing	ashen rock salt
blue-green	a green jade emblem of rank	dark-blue indigo
yellow	bright yellow gauze	soil from the Yellow River
black	a double layer of lacquer	dullish grey earth

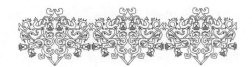

2. The Bright-lit Hall, the Physiognomy of Face

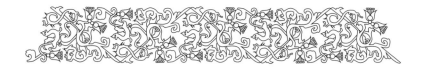

明堂者, 鼻也, 闕者, 眉間也, 庭者, 顏也.

蕃者, 頰側也, 蔽者, 耳門也, 其間欲方大去之十步.

皆見於外, 如是者壽, 必中百歲.

THE BRIGHT-LIT HALL AT COURT is at the nose;

The lookout tower by the main gate is the space between the
   eyebrows;

The courtyard is the high space above.

Where are the hedges? Either side at the cheeks.

Where are the side-screens? At the opening out of the ears.

The whole area between them should be square and large, viewed
   from a distance of ten paces.

When all this is seen on the outside, your life will attain one
   hundred years.

Li Zhongzi: If at ten paces these areas are clearly visible outside they are
obviously 'square and large'.

明堂骨高以起平以直, 五臟次於中央, 六腑挾其兩側.

首面上於闕庭, 王宮在於下極.

The 'bright-lit hall' starts at the upper bones of the face,

Reaching out horizontally and the same on both sides.

The five *zang* are arrayed in the central region of the face; the six
   fu positioned on either side.

105

The head and face lie above at the 'lookout tower' – by the main
   gate leading to the courtyard.
The 'imperial palace' is positioned immediately below.

五臟安於胸中, 真色以致.
病色不見, 明堂潤澤以清.
If the five *zang* are safe within the chest.
Their true colours are brought out.
The colour of sickness is not seen
And the 'bright-lit hall' is glisteningly clear.

Li Zhongzi: The climates of the five *zang* are all shown in the central region of
the face; the climates of the six *fu* along the four sides.

五色之見也, 各出其色部.
部骨陷者, 必不免於病矣. 其色部乘襲者, 雖病甚, 不死矣.
Each of the colours is seen, coming out at its own region.
If any colour is seen sunken into a region of the bone, you will
   not escape sickness.
If any colour is riding over and invading into a region,
Then although the sickness is severe, it will not prove fatal.

青黑為痛, 黃赤為熱, 白為寒.
Greeny-blue and black mean pain,
Yellow and red mean fever,
White means cold.

其色麤以明, 沉夭者為甚.
其色上行者, 病益甚,
其色下行, 如雲徹散者, 病方已.
A colour which is strongly toned signifies brightness,
A colour drained out or dried up signifies severity.
A colour mounting upwards means the sickness is worsening,
A colour travelling downward, like a cloud dispersing, signifies
   the sickness is already over.

五色各有臟部, 有外部有內部也,
色從外部走內部者, 其病從外走內,
其色從內走外者, 其病從內走外.

Each of the 'five colours' has its own *zang* region;
There are outer regions and inner regions.
If a colour runs from an outer to an inner region, the sickness is
    running from out to within.
If the colour runs from an inner to an outer region, the sickness is
    running from in to without.

病生於內者, 先治其陰, 後治其陽, 反者益甚,
其病生於陽者, 先治其外, 後治其內, 反者益甚.

If the sickness starts within, first treat the Yin and later the Yang.
If you reverse this, it will worsen.
If the sickness starts in the Yang, first treat the outer and then the
    inner.
If you reverse this, it will worsen.

常候闕中, 薄澤為風, 沖濁為痺, 在地為厥.
此其常也, 各以其色言其病.

Always attend to the 'lookout tower' by the main gate.
If the colour is much reduced and dampish, it signifies wind;
If it appears infused and dirty, it signifies *bi* immobility,
If it appears in the 'land region', it means weakening.
These are the usual deductions – in each case the colour identifies
    the sickness.

Li Zhongzi: Weakening or 'reversing' 厥 *jue* ailments are due to the vicissitudes
of cold and damp. These sicknesses begin below. Hence the colour is first
present in the 'land region'. This is a term used among face-readers for the
'land pavilion' or chin.

大氣入於臟腑者, 不病而卒死矣.
赤色出兩顴, 大如拇指者, 病雖小愈, 必卒死.
黑色出於庭, 大如拇指, 必不病而卒死.

When a great energy enters the organs, there may be no sign of
    sickness but eventually you die.

When a red colour comes out on both cheeks, as large as a thumb,
You sicken and although you may recover a little, eventually you
    die.
When a black colour comes out at the 'courtyard', as large as a
    thumb,
There will be no sign of sickness, but eventually you die.

Zhang Jiebin: A 'great energy' signifies a great malign *xie* energy.

庭者, 首面也, 闕上者, 咽喉也, 闕中者, 肺也, 下極者, 心也.
直下者, 肝也, 肝左者, 膽也, 下者, 脾也.

The 'courtyard' corresponds to the head and face.
Above the 'lookout tower' to the main gate is the throat.
Within the 'lookout tower' to the main gate lie the lungs.
At a lower extreme is the heart, directly below is the liver.
What is left of the liver? The gallbladder.
What is below? The spleen.

方上者, 胃也, 中央者, 大腸也, 挾大腸者, 腎也, 當腎者, 臍也.
面王以上者, 小腸也, 面王以下者, 膀胱子處也.

What is located at the 'upper aspects'? The stomach.
What are located in the 'middle regions'? The large intestines.
What are located beside the large intestines? The kidneys.
What is before the kidneys? The navel.
What are located above the 'monarch of the face'?
The small intestines.
What are located beneath the 'monarch of the face'?
The bladder and 'child residence'.

Li Zhongzi: The 'monarch of the face' means the tip of the nose. 'Child residence' is a name for the uterus. The area of the 'middle of man' acupoint (*renzhong* Du 26, at the philtrum) being smooth, shallow and hairless in men usually indicates no offspring. It is the same in women. When the 'middle of man' is deep and broad, they tend to have easy confinements.

顴者, 肩也, 顴後者, 臂也, 臂下者, 手也, 目內眥上者, 膺乳也, 挾繩而上者,
    背也.

What are the high bones of the cheeks? The shoulders.

What are back from the high bones on the cheeks? The arms.
What are located beneath the arms? The hands.
What are located in the upper inner corners of the eyes?
The bosom and breast.
What is above, either side, in the 'cord areas'? The back.

Li Zhongzi: The 'cord areas' describe the outer cheek where the cords from a hat hang down.

循牙車以下者, 股也. 中央者, 膝也.
膝以下者, 脛也. 當脛以下者, 足也.
巨分者, 股裏也, 巨屈者, 膝臏也.

Following the line of the 'tooth carriage' below, you come to the
    thighs.
Its central region corresponds to the knees.
Below the knees are the shinbones.
Beneath the shinbones are the feet.
The 'large split' in the face corresponds to the inner thigh;
The 'large bend' corresponds to the kneecap.

Li Zhongzi: The 'tooth carriage' is the jawbone. The 'large split' describes the wide creases either side of the mouth. The 'large bend' is the angled bone at the bottom of the cheek.

此五臟六腑肢節之部也, 各有部分 —
有部分, 用陰和陽, 用陽和陰, 當明部分, 萬舉萬當.

Each of the *zangfu*, limbs and tendons has its own special region –
And in each you should use Yin to harmonise Yang and Yang to
    harmonise Yin.
Clearly make an effort to know each special region,
And ten thousand attempts will mean every one successful.

Li Zhongzi: Once each separate region is clearly known and if Yin and Yang are not healthy, then if the Yang is overbearing, stimulate Yin – taking Yin to harmonise Yang; and if the Yin is cold then tonify the fire – taking Yang to harmonise Yin. Thenceforth if you clearly know each special region and apply these methods of treatment, in ten thousand attempts, every one of them will prove successful.

能別左右, 是謂大道.
男女異位, 故曰陰陽.
審察澤夭, 謂之良工.

If you are able to distinguish left and right,
This is what is meant by 'great technique'.
Male and female have different positions,
So then Yin and Yang are mentioned.
To inspect the dampish or drying out –
May be called 'supreme craftsmanship'!

沉濁為內, 浮澤為外.

A colour draining or dirty means an illness within,
Being puffy or dampish means an illness without.

黃赤為風, 青黑為痛, 白為寒, 黃而膏.

Yellow and red mean wind,
Greeny-blue and black mean pain,
White means cold, yellow means pus.

潤為膿, 赤甚者為血. 痛甚為攣, 寒甚為皮不仁.

A moistening colour refers to the vessels,
Extreme red signifies blood.
If the pain is severe, it makes for twitching,
If the cold is severe, the skin becomes numb.

五色各見其部, 察其浮沉, 以知淺深, 察其澤夭, 以觀成敗,
察其散搏, 以知遠近, 視色上下, 以知病處.

As each of the five colours is seen in its region:
Examine whether it is puffy or draining and you know the depth
    of the sickness;
Examine whether dampish or dried out and you can see whether
    there will be success or failure;
Examine whether it is breaking up or gathering and you know
    whether the illness is distant or near;
Examine whether the colour is above and below, and you know
    the location of the disease.

Li Zhongzi: If the colour is breaking up and not contained, the illness is near. If it is gathering and not breaking up, the illness is still distant.

色明不麤, 沉夭為甚; 不明不澤, 其病不甚.
If the hue is not strongly toned, but draining or dried out, the
   sickness is severe;
But if the hue is not bright, or not dampish, the sickness is not
   necessarily severe.

其色散, 駒駒然, 未有聚. 其病散而氣痛, 聚未成也.
If the colour breaks up like a frisking foal, the sickness is not yet
   contained.
If the sickness breaks up and it creates pain, it means the
   containment is not successful.

腎乘心, 心先病, 腎為應: 色皆如是.
When the kidneys encroach on the heart, the heart is first sick but
   the kidneys show a response:
All the other colours act in this same way.

Li Zhongzi: The heart is first sick within, but the kidneys show a colour which is the response outside – for instance, black seen at the lower extremity of the face.

男子色在於面王, 為小腹痛, 下為卵痛.
其圜直為莖痛, 高為本, 下為首, 狐疝痛陰之屬也.
In a male, if the colour is situated at the 'monarch of the face', it
   means pain in the lower belly,
Reaching down to make the testicles ache.

Rounded or square, it means the penis aches.
If the colour is high up it means the root of the penis;
If it is low down it means the head.
These suggest problems like inguinal hernias or painful sex organs.

Li Zhongzi: 'Rounded or straight' refers to the 'water spring' acupoint (another name for 'middle of man', Du 26). This point has a border which can either be rounded or straight…'high up' or 'low down' refers to higher or lower parts of this area.

女子在於面王, 為膀胱子處之病.

散為痛, 搏為聚. 方員左右, 各如其色形.

In a female, if the colour is situated at the 'monarch of the face', it means a sickness of the bladder or uterus.

Breaking up means pain,

Gathering together means being contained.

Whatever its shape, left or right –

Each time the colour shows the shape of the disease.

其隨而下至胝, 為淫, 有潤如膏狀, 為暴食不潔.

When it follows on down to the very bottom of the face, it means insidious pollution;

When it looks moist and greasy, it means a fierce appetite for newly prepared food.

Here the whole face is seen as an entrance or gateway into the imperial court or 'temple' of the body. The *zangfu* organs and limbs are arrayed on the face – just as they are arrayed in the body. This remarkable document details how watching the location, spread, intensity and movement of colours on the face shows the state of the body within. It states clearly that 'if the five *zang* are safe within the chest, their true colours are brought out'.

These picturesque verses relate the facial regions to the rest of the body. They describe the character of the colour as it changes and moves, and the implications for disease. If the five *zang* are safe, their proper colours appear; if the colours appear sunken and ride over or invade another region, it is unfavourable. Attend to the 'lookout tower', the space between the eyebrows, and also to the 'bright-lit hall' by the nose and upper bones of the face, reaching out horizontally to both sides – here are relayed messages relevant to health. Supreme craftsmanship communicates with this area. Is the area dampish or drying out, sinking or scattering, and so on? Through contrasting and combining such signs, and examining the pulse, you decide their lot of life and death. This text is invaluable. Mostly it indicates the progression of disease – a few lines signify the return of health. The text has been fairly altered by editors, notably Huang Fumi. I mostly follow the NJZY.

PHYSIOGNOMY OF FACE

the bright-lit hall	upper bones of the face
the lookout tower by the main gate	space between the eyebrows
the courtyard	the high space above
the hedges	either side of the cheeks
the side screens	the opening out of the ears

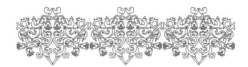

3. The Basis of Health in the Face

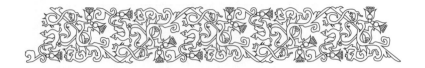

面黃目青, 面黃目赤, 面黃目白, 面黃目黑者, 皆不死也.
面青目赤, 面赤目白, 面青目黑, 面黑目白, 面赤目青, 皆死也.

THE FACE YELLOW, around the eyes blue-green,
The face yellow, around the eyes red,
The face yellow, around the eyes white,
The face yellow, around the eyes black,
These are all not fatal.

The face blue-green, around the eyes red,
The face red, around the eyes white,
The face green, around the eyes black,
The face black, around the eyes white,
The face red, around the eyes green,
These are all fatal.

Li Zhongzi: Yellow is the proper colour of the 'central region' of the soil. The *wuxing* take the soil as foundation. If the stomach qi is still present, the condition is not fatal. When there is no yellow in the complexion, the stomach qi is finished and comes to an end. Hence all the above conditions are fatal.

As a basis for health, the idea of equity between Yin and Yang is quite easy to understand. Here it is represented by the quality of yellowness in the face. The character for 'yellow' 黃 *huang* stands, of course, for balance. As Li Zhongzi indicates, 'yellow' stands for the central element of the *wuxing*; that is, the soil. As wood, fire, metal and water stand for east, south, west and north respectively, so the central soil (earth) represents the ubiquity of the land. The care given to their soils by the Chinese is well testified. It is possible to read 死 *si* as 'extreme' or 'deteriorating' here, rather than 'fatal' – lessening the punch of the text.

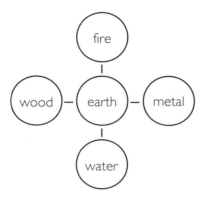

A basic *wuxing* diagram

Xue Shengbai comments on this chapter:

> Gazing at the colour, listening, questioning and cutting into the beat of the pulse, these are what are called 'the four examinations'. But gazing at the colour is foremost among the four examinations. Never by solely relying on a single pulse is it possible to effect a treatment. The *Neijing* says: 'When cutting into the beat of the pulse, in all circumstances, you should also observe the clarity of light, distinguishing among the five colours to see which of the five *zang* have excess or not enough, which of the six *fu* are strong or failing, and the fullness or weakness of the physical body. ' By this process of contrasting and combining you may decide their lot of life and death. There are many sayings concerning colour: 'If body and energies agree together, it means they can be cured'; 'If the colour is damp or puffy it means it will easily end'; 'If pulse and colour can be combined, anything is possible', and so on.

FATALITY IN THE FACE AND EYES

the face	around the eyes	outcome
yellow	blue-green	not fatal
yellow	red	not fatal
yellow	white	not fatal
yellow	black	not fatal
blue-green	red	fatal
red	white	fatal
green	black	fatal
black	white	fatal
red	green	fatal

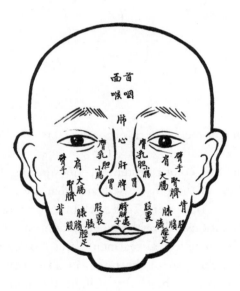

Picture of the human face displaying the *zangfu*

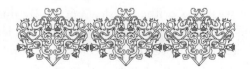

Questions for Review of Chapter III

1. How is the body's Yang purity shown in the facial complexion? Describe *in a few words* the particular qualities of sickness when it is shown on the face.

2. Draw a simple diagram of the face and show the rough location of the 'main gate'; 'bright-lit hall'; 'side screens'; and 'courtyard'.

3. Describe briefly the significance of colour when it is changing or moving on the face.

4. Why is the quality of 'yellowness' important in the facial complexion?

Characters in Chapter III

purity and brightness 夫精明 *jingming*

glistening 潤澤 *runze*

bright-lit hall 明堂 *mingtang*

weakening or reversing ailments 厥 *jue*

yellow (complexion) 黃 *huang*

fatal, extreme, deteriorating 死 *si*

IV

The Quiet Pulse

What my heart understands, my mouth cannot
proclaim…if we are not acquainted with the
rough, how can we sift out the smooth!

Key Ideas

1. *The Method of the Pulse Exam*
   the quiet exam, the pulse at fault, both colour and pulse
   involved, purity and brightness, pulse positions, contrasting
   and combining the signs

2. *If a Single Pulse Stands Out*
   the lone pulse, sickness

3. *The Primacy of the Pulse*
   the precedence of the pulse

4. *In Attending to the Pulse*
   the art of the pulse, be humbled, depth, its seasonal character

5. *In Spring, the Pulse is in the Liver*
   seasonal variation, excess and insufficiency, sickness,
   symptomology, the unique quality of the spleen pulse

6. *The Healthy, Sick and Fatal Pulses*
   characters of the healthy, sick and fatal pulses

7. *The Arrival of the Fatal Pulse*
   characters of the fatal pulse, conferring incapacity, how to time fatality

8. *The Ultimate Tool*
   colour and pulse, negligence, a return to the real people of old

9. *A Common Fault in the Pulse Exam*
   the rough, hasty or sloppy exam

Some questions for review can be found at the end of this chapter.

1. The Method of the Pulse Exam

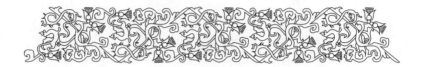

診法常以平旦, 陰氣未動, 陽氣未散.

飲食未進, 經脈未盛. 絡脈調勻, 氣血未亂. 故乃可診有過之脈.

THE METHOD OF EXAMINATION is regularly done at dawn.

When the Yin qi has not yet stirred and the Yang qi not yet scattered,

Food and drink have not yet been taken, and the main channels not yet filled.

The subsidiary channels are attuned and the qi and blood not yet distributed.

At that moment you must diagnose which pulse is at fault.

Li Zhongzi: In the body the nutrient and defensive qi travels by day in the Yang, and by night in the Yin. Then at dawn both meet up at the 'inch-wide mouth' at the wrist. Thus the pulse exam ought to be regularly done at dawn.

Zhang Jiebin: The hour of dawn is the connecting-point of Yin and Yang. Yang commands the day, Yin commands the night. Yang commands without, Yin commands within. 'At fault' means the pulse has not found its mean position, but slipped off.

Ma Shi: In general, people have disease – just as in any affair, mistakes are made. This is why the text mentions the pulse 'at fault'. The whole of the *Neijing* was written to protect against this.

切脈動靜而視精明.

察五色, 觀五臟有餘不足, 六腑強弱, 形之盛衰.

以此參伍, 決死生之分.

When you cut into the beat of the pulse, look also into the purity
  in the eyes.

Examine the 'five colours' and observe which of the 'five *zang*' has
  excess or not enough;

And then see which of the 'six *fu*' is working or failing,

And whether the body is strong or in decline.

Thereby by contrasting and combining these signs

You may decide their lot of life and death.

Li Zhongzi: Look at the 'five colours' and you observe the weakness or strength
of the organs; inspect the physical body and you determine whether the
sickness is filling or failing.

Wu Kun: Within the eye lies the pupil – it shows the activity of the mind.

Zhang Jiebin: Picking up three differing things is 'combining' them, taking up
five of the same kind is 'contrasting' them; in general this and that reflect each
other, difference and sameness show linked symptoms – which means we
have a special need to work out carefully all the detail. Just as the *Yijing* states:
'Contrast and combine (*canwu*) the changes…pick up the main threads of the
count and you will begin to understand. '

Hua Shou: Use pulse and colour, *zang* and *fu*, body and qi – combine them
together, put them down, contrast them, then lay them out straight!

尺內兩旁則季脅也, 尺外以候腎, 尺裏以候腹中.

附上左外以候肝, 內以候鬲, 右外以候胃, 內以候脾.

上附上右外以候肺, 內以候胸中. 左外以候心, 內以候膻中.

The 'inner foot' position, both sides, shows the pattern of the
  floating ribs.

The 'outer foot' position may be used to attend to the kidneys,

The 'inner foot' position may be used to attend to the belly.

Attached in front, at the outer left, you may attend to the liver,

While within, you may attend to the diaphragm.

On the outer right you may attend to the stomach,

While within, you may attend to the spleen.

In front of this and attached in front, on the outer right you may
   attend to the lungs –
While within, you may attend to the 'middle chest'.
On the outer left you may attend to the heart –
While within, you may attend to the middle of the chest.

This chapter contains some of the most evocative images in the
whole of the *Neijing*. They are used to evoke the sense of harmony
or disharmony felt at the wrist pulse. This section explains how
you need quiet to conduct a proper examination. Dawn is the
best time, when the Yin (confusion) of the day has not yet
stirred and the Yang (new life) not yet scattered. The position,
depth and quality of the pulse is *just as* important as, if not *more*
important than, the rate. I have appended Li Zhongzi's excellent
commentaries below to make the verses clear. This being said, in
pulse diagnosis, as in colour, there is ample scope for an individual
view. The diagnosis of the pulse tests, to the utmost, a physician's
discipline of mind and sensitivity.

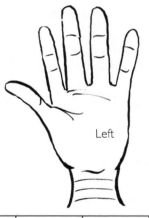
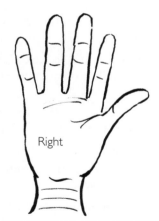

Left   Right

'foot' to 'inch' ⬆	outer	within		within	outer	'foot' to 'inch' ⬆
	heart	middle chest		middle chest	lungs	
	liver	diaphragm		spleen	stomach	
	kidneys	floating ribs		floating ribs	kidneys	

Wrist diagram of the pulses

Mencius, the Confucian philosopher, said: 'In retaining a man, look at the pupils of his eyes! If he is true to himself, the pupils are bright and clear. ' This chapter follows directly on the heels of the colour chapter and, indeed, since ancient times colour and pulse have been entwined in diagnosis. As the text says, 'When you cut into the beat of the pulse, look also into the purity in the eyes. ' To 'decide their lot of life and death' is a telling phrase. Zhang Jiebin explains 'to contrast and combine' 參伍 *canwu* rather enigmatically – 'this and that reflect each other, difference and sameness show linked symptoms': the term *canwu* is drawn from the all-encompassing 'Grand Appendix' or *Zici* to the *Yijing* – where it explains the laying out of the yarrow-stalks in divination. Certainly the boundary between the occult and the medical has often been unclear, even in present-day China. To *canwu* in diagnosis in order to reach a conclusion means to contrast, that is, not to arrange uniformly – and then to combine. Not to arrange uniformly is to 'contrast' – so separate out their differences; to divide into groups of similars is to 'combine'. This term illustrates accurately the *yinyang* of the human mind, as it travels towards a solution.

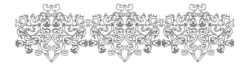

2. If a Single Pulse Stands Out

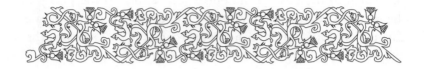

獨小者病, 獨大者病, 獨疾者病, 獨遲者病,
獨熱者病, 獨寒者病, 獨陷下者病.

ONE ON ITS OWN IS SMALL, there is sickness,
One on its own is large, there is sickness,
One on its own is fast, there is sickness,
One on its own is slow, there is sickness,
One on its own is hot, there is sickness,
One on its own is cold, there is sickness,
One on its own, sunken, there is sickness.

First there must be normalcy within the pulse. If a reading is made at one of the pulse positions and a single pulse stands out – on its own, small or large, fast or slow, hot or cold, or even sunken – there must be an imbalance, and therefore sickness. When taking the pulse, look for harmony.

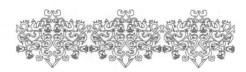

3. The Primacy of the Pulse

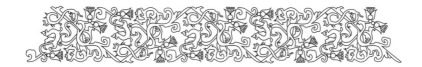

形氣有餘, 脈氣不足死.
脈氣有餘, 形氣不足生.

IF THE QI OF THE PHYSICAL BODY is in surplus
But the qi of the pulse is insufficient, it will prove fatal.
If the qi of the pulse is surplus
But the qi of the body is insufficient,
It means you will survive.

When investigating the pulse, we should also look at how the body presents. Even if someone appears weakened, or wasted, if the pulse has a surplus of energy, the patient will survive. It is the inner presentation that counts. The pulse carries the body, not the body which carries the pulse.

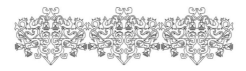

4. In Attending to the Pulse

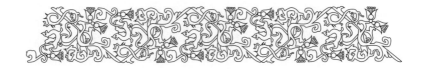

持脈有道, 虛靜為保.

THERE IS AN ART IN ATTENDING TO THE PULSE.
Be humbled, quiet and guarded.

春日浮, 如魚之游在波, 夏日在膚, 泛泛乎萬物有餘.
秋日下膚, 蟄蟲將去, 冬日在骨, 蟄蟲周密, 君子居室.

On spring days the pulse is 'floating',
Like a fish suspended in the eddy of a stream;
On summer days the pulse lies at the skin,
Floating freely, everything in surplus.
On autumn days it lies under the skin,
Like a torpid insect ready to creep away.
On winter days it lies at the bone,
Like a torpid insect, totally hidden –
Just as the *junzi* stays hidden at home.

故曰, 知內者按而紀之, 知外者終而始之, 此六者持脈之大法.

Therefore, as is said:
'You know them within, press down and record them.
You know them without, determine their beginning and end. '
These are the six rules which form the supreme principle in
    attending to the pulse.

Li Zhongzi: 'Within' means the *zang*'s qi; the *zang* are represented in position
so you can 'press down and record them'. 'Without' means the channel's qi;
the channels are in a set sequence so you can 'determine their beginning and
end'. Be clear on the six rules – the four seasonal qi energies, within and

without – and all sickness, internal and external, Yin and Yang will be sorted and understood. This is why these six rules are the supreme principle for attending to the pulse.

The art in attending to the pulse is to be quiet in manner and guarded in approach. The spring pulse should be 'floating', like a fish suspended in a stream; in the middle of the year the pulse is 'at the skin', relishing the summer warmth; on autumn days it retreats 'under the skin', like a torpid insect 'ready to creep away'; and on winter days it sinks like stone, almost lying 'at the bone' – totally hidden. For Li Zhongzi and Zhang Jiebin the six rules are 'the four seasonal qi energies, within and without'. There are other interpretations.

THE PULSE

on spring days	floating	a fish suspended in the eddy of a stream
on summer days	at the skin	floating freely, everything in surplus
on autumn days	under the skin	a torpid insect ready to creep away
on winter days	at the bone	a torpid insect, totally hidden

5. In Spring, the Pulse is in the Liver

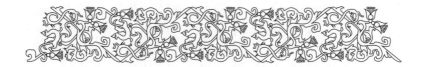

春脈者, 肝也, 東方木也, 萬物之所以始生也.
故其氣來軟弱, 輕虛而滑.
端直以長, 故曰弦, 反此者病.

IN SPRING, THE PULSE IS IN THE LIVER; and in 'wood'
    from an easterly direction,
Whereby all myriad things have their beginning and birth.
Its qi is pliable and weak when arriving –
Slightly empty and slippery.
It is upright, and extending itself;
Thus the pulse is 'stretched as a cord'.
To arrive contrary to this is sickness.

其氣來實而強, 此謂太過, 病在外.
其氣來不實而微, 此謂不及, 病在中.
太過則令人善忘, 忽忽眩冒而巔疾.
其不及, 則令人胸痛引背, 下則兩脅胠滿.

If the qi arrives solidly and strong,
This means excess and the sickness is without;
If the qi arrives not strong but minute,
It means insufficiency and the sickness is within.
If there is excess, people tend to be forgetful;
All of a sudden they become dizzy,
Their sight fails and they suffer bouts of madness.

If there is insufficiency the chest aches, leading into the back,
And both flanks below feel swollen and full.

夏脈者心也, 南方火也, 萬物之所以盛長也.
故其氣來盛去衰, 故曰鉤, 反此者病.

In summer, the pulse is in the heart; and in 'fire' from a southerly
    direction,
Whereby all myriad things fill out and grow.
Its qi is full when arriving but fades when departing –
And thus termed 'slightly hooked'.
To arrive contrary to this is sickness.

其氣來盛去亦盛, 此謂太過, 病在外,
其氣來不盛去反盛, 此謂不及, 病在中.
太過則令人身熱而膚痛, 為浸淫,
其不及則令人煩心, 上見咳唾, 下為氣泄.

If the qi arrives full but also departs full,
This means excess and the sickness is without;
If the qi arrives not full but instead departs full,
It means insufficiency and the sickness is within.
If there is excess, the body is hot and the skin and flesh painful –
So it means there is insidious pollution.
If there is insufficiency it makes for anxiety in the heart;
You see spittle coughed up above,
While below it creates diarrhoea.

秋脈者, 肺也, 西方金也, 萬物之所以收成也.
故其氣來輕虛以浮, 來急去散, 故曰浮, 反此者病.

In autumn, the pulse is in the lungs; and in 'metal' from a
    westerly direction,
Whereby all myriad things find closure and completion.
Its qi is slightly empty when arriving and floating.
It arrives hurriedly and departs scattering, thus it is termed
    'floating'.
To arrive contrary to this is sickness.

其氣來毛而中央堅, 兩傍虛, 此謂太過, 病在外.
其氣來毛而微, 此謂不及, 病在中.
太過則令人逆氣而背痛, 慍慍然,
其不及則令人喘, 呼吸少氣而咳, 上氣見血, 下聞病音.

If the qi arrives 'feathery' but hard in the central region and weak
  at both sides,
This means excess and the sickness is without;
If the qi arrives 'feathery' and minute,
It means insufficiency and the sickness is within.
If the qi is in excess, people have a rebellious nature and back
  pain,
They feel worried and are depressed.
If there is insufficiency they have difficulty in breathing,
There is shortness of breath and coughing;
They bring up blood above, while below the sickness makes a
  sound.

冬脈者, 腎也, 北方水也, 萬物之所以含藏也.
故其氣來沈以搏, 故曰營, 反此者病.

In winter, the pulse is in the kidneys; and in 'water' from a
  northerly direction,
Whereby all myriad things lie in together and are dormant.
Its qi arrives from deep within and strikes out at the finger;
Thus the pulse is termed 'fenced in'.
To arrive contrary to this is sickness.

其氣來如彈石者, 此謂太過, 病在外,
其去如數者, 此謂不及, 病在中.
太過則令人解㑊, 脊脈痛, 而少氣不欲言.
其不及則令人心懸, 如病飢, 䏚中清, 脊中痛, 少腹滿, 小便變.

If the qi arrives like a flung stone,
This means excess and the sickness is without;
If the qi departs rapidly,
It means insufficiency and the sickness is within.
If the qi is in excess, people tend to feel idle;
While the vessels down the spine ache,

They are short of breath and do not want to speak.
If there is insufficiency they imagine a feeling inside like hunger;
The flanks below feel light and empty,
There is an aching in the spine, the lower belly feels full,
And the urine changes colour.

脾脈者土也, 孤臟, 以灌四傍者也.
善者不可得見, 惡者可見.
The spleen pulse is that of the earth.
It is the solitary *zang* organ which irrigates all four sides.
When it functions well it cannot be seen,
When it functions badly it can be seen.

其來如水之流者, 此謂太過, 病在外.
如鳥之喙者, 此謂不及, 病在中.
If it arrives like rushing water,
It means excess and the sickness is without,
If it arrives like a pecking crow,
Then the qi is insufficient and the sickness is within.

Note the careful description again given to the pulse in each season. Spring: the pulse is 'slightly empty and slippery, upright and extending itself'; summer: the pulse is 'full when arriving, but fades when departing'; autumn: the pulse remains 'slightly empty when arriving and floating, arrives hurriedly and departs scattering'; while in winter, the pulse 'arrives from deep within and strikes out at the finger'. In spring it should be slightly stretched, in summer slightly hooked, in autumn slightly floating, and in winter slightly fenced in. We can be reminded of the movement of 'birth and growth, closure and storage' given in Chapter I, Section 4, 'The Rhythm of the Seasons'. As the pulse departs from the 'norm', in 'excess' or in 'insufficiency', so there occur the conditions for disease. Note also the uniqueness of the spleen pulse, representing the 'earth'. When it functions well, it 'cannot be seen'; when it functions badly, it can be seen. This echoes the image in *Laozi* 11 of the cartwheel turning on a hub: 'thirty spokes come together in the hub, but it is what is not there that enables the carriage to be used'; and of the building of a room, 'cut doors and windows to make a room, and it is what is not there that enables a room to be used'. In other words, emptiness enables power: as the empty centre of the wheel means the carriage can be moved – and open doors and windows bring in light and utility to a room. I follow entirely the editing of the NJZY for this important chapter.

THE SEASONAL PULSE

spring	liver	wood	easterly	beginning and birth	'stretched as a cord'	pliable and weak when arriving, slightly empty and slippery
summer	heart	fire	southerly	fill out and grow	'slightly hooked'	full when arriving but fades when departing
autumn	lungs	metal	westerly	closure and completion	'floating'	empty when arriving hurried and departs scattering
winter	kidneys	water	northerly	lying in and dormant	'fenced in'	arrives from deep and strikes out at the finger

6. The Healthy, Sick and Fatal Pulses

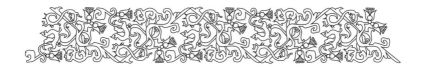

夫平心脈來, 累累如連珠, 如循琅玕, 曰心平. 夏以胃氣為本.

AT THE ARRIVAL OF THE HEALTHY PULSE of the heart,
    the beats are continuous, one following another –
Like pearls strung on a string,
Like a necklace made of smooth reddish jade stones.
This is the 'healthy pulse of the heart'.
In summer it takes the stomach qi as root.

病心脈來, 喘喘連屬, 其中微曲, 曰心病.
死心脈來, 前曲後居, 如操帶鉤, 曰心死.

The arrival of the sick pulse of the heart is tortuous, each beat
    joined to the other but slightly kinked in.
This is the sick pulse of the heart.
The arrival of the fatal pulse of the heart is kinked in front while
    held back behind,
As if caught by a belt buckle.
This is the fatal pulse of the heart.

Li Zhongzi: 'Pearls strung on a string' and 'reddish jade stones' are similes for being full to the brim, smooth and glistening; as if slightly fastened with a buckle, with the stomach qi as root.

Li Zhongzi: 'Tortuous, each beat joined to the other' is the image of a rapid, fast beat; 'slightly kinked in' means the kink is more and the stomach qi less.

Li Zhongzi: 'Kinked in front' means that when lightly pressed on it becomes hard and grows larger; 'held back behind' means that when pressed on it feels penned in and solid, as if there were a buckle restraining a belt. The significance of this is that it is wholly out of good harmony.

平肺脈來, 厭厭聶聶, 如落榆莢, 曰肺平. 秋以胃氣為本.

The arrival of the healthy pulse of the lung is slightly crushed in
    and as if delicate –
Like an elm seed dropping to the ground.
This is the 'healthy pulse of the lung'.
In the autumn it takes the stomach qi as root.

病肺脈來, 不上不下, 如循雞羽, 曰肺病.
死肺脈來, 如物之浮, 如風吹毛, 曰肺死.

The arrival of the sick pulse of the lung has nothing either above
    or below.
It is like stroking the hand along a chicken's feather.
This is the sick pulse of the lung.
The arrival of the fatal lung pulse is like brushing your fingers
    against a floating object,
Like feathers blown in the wind.
This is the fatal pulse of the lung.

Li Zhongzi: 'Slightly crushed in and as if delicate' is the image of being uneven; 'an elm seed dropping to the ground' is the image of being feathery; lightly floating in a relaxed manner means it has stomach qi.

Li Zhongzi: 'Having nothing either above or below' again means the pulse is uneven; 'like stroking the hand along a chicken's feather' again means something feathery – but the featheriness is more and the stomach qi less.

Li Zhongzi: 'Like brushing your fingers against a floating object' means the pulse has no foundation; 'like feathers blown in the wind' means it is scattered and truly confused. There is only the featheriness without any stomach qi.

平肝脈來, 軟弱招招, 如揭長竿末梢, 曰肝平. 春以胃氣為本.

The arrival of the healthy pulse of the liver is pliable, supple and
    beckoning –
Like the tip of a raised bamboo cane.
This is the 'healthy pulse of the liver'.
In spring it takes the stomach qi as root.

病肝脈來, 盈實而滑, 如循長竿, 曰肝病.

死肝脈來, 急益勁如新張弓弦, 曰肝死.

The arrival of the sick pulse of the liver is full and substantial, but
    also slippery;

It is like the obvious movement of a long bamboo cane.

This is the sick pulse of the liver.

The arrival of the fatal liver pulse is hurried,

With added tension, like the cord of a newly strung bow.

This is the fatal pulse of the liver.

Li Zhongzi: 'Beckoning' means as if from far off; 'raised' means lifted up like a
long raised bamboo cane. The pulse must be pliant, like the slightly slack cord
of a bow. The cord is springy and has stomach qi.

Li Zhongzi: 'Full and substantial, but also slippery' means it is sprung too much,
a cane is mentioned, but not its tip, losing the idea of 'springiness'. Now the
cord is more, the stomach qi less.

Li Zhongzi: 'Tension' implies being forceful and hurried. The cord is stretched
excessively. There is only the 'cord' without the stomach qi.

平脾脈來, 和柔相離, 如雞踐地, 曰脾平. 長夏以胃氣為本.

The arrival of the healthy pulse of the spleen is soft and gentle,
    each beat divided from the next –

Like a chicken treading the earth.

This is the 'healthy pulse of the spleen'.

In late summer it takes the stomach qi as root.

病脾病來, 實而盈數, 如雞舉足, 曰脾病.

死脾脈來, 銳堅如鳥之喙, 如鳥之距, 如屋之漏, 如水之流, 曰脾死.

The arrival of the sick pulse of the spleen is substantial, full and
    fast,

Like a chicken picking up its foot.

This is the sick pulse of the spleen.

The arrival of the fatal spleen pulse is sharp and hard like the bill
    of a bird, or a cock's spur,

Like a roof letting in the rain, or a stream bursting its banks.

This is the fatal pulse of the spleen.

Li Zhongzi: 'Soft and gentle', it sounds close but reaches afar…each beat 'divided from the next' means each beat is clearly distinct. It is like a chicken treading the earth, slowly and unhurriedly, the marvel of the stomach qi.

Li Zhongzi: 'Substantial, full and fast' means forceful, hurried and no longer soft. The chicken is picking up her front foot. Now the weakness is more, the stomach qi less.

Li Zhongzi: 'Like the bill of a bird' means forcibly; 'a cock's spur' means hurriedly; 'a roof letting in the rain' means confusion; 'a stream bursting its banks' means scattered. The spleen qi has already gone.

平腎脈來, 喘喘累累如鉤, 按之而堅, 曰腎平. 冬以胃氣為本.

The arrival of the healthy pulse of the kidney is tortuous but
   continuous –
As if caught by a belt buckle.
Press down on it and it feels hard.
This is the 'healthy pulse of the kidney'.
In winter it takes the stomach qi as root.

病腎脈來如引葛, 按之益堅, 曰腎病.
死腎脈來發如奪索, 辟辟石彈石, 曰腎死.

The arrival of the sick pulse of the kidney is like drawing down on
   a creeper.
Press down on it and it becomes even harder.
This is the sick pulse of the kidney.
The arrival of the fatal kidney pulse is like tugging on a long rope,
   or a far-flung stone.
This is the fatal pulse of the kidney.

Li Zhongzi: 'Tortuous but continuous, as if caught by a belt buckle', both describe the Yang pulse of the heart. Together with there being the sense of a 'stone' when pressed on deeply, this means Yin and Yang are in good harmony. The kidney pulse retains some stomach qi.

Li Zhongzi: 'Drawing down on a creeper' is like dragging something out continuously, getting it all tangled and muddled up – you press your finger down on it and it becomes even harder. The 'stone' is more, the stomach qi less.

Li Zhongzi: When a long rope is tugged between two people it becomes taut and full of tension; a 'far-flung stone' means there is only the feeling of a 'stone', with no stomach qi.

These evocative verses beautifully describe the pulse qualities: this time listed by *zang* organ, each pulse illustrated – in its healthy, sick and fatal manner. The passing beat may be felt as a necklace, or chain of smooth pebbles or stones, as if caught up by a buckle; or as an elm seed dropping to the ground, or as feathers blown in the wind; like the beckoning tip of a raised bamboo cane, or the tight cord of a newly strung bow; like a chicken cautiously picking up its feet, or hard as a cock's spur, and so on. The pulse of each organ takes a single season of the year 'as root'. The general characteristic of a sick or fatal pulse is that it departs from the norm. In other words, the beat needs to be soft, but not too soft, and firm, but not too firm. Compare *Laozi* 77: 'Is not Nature's Way just like the stringing of a bow? What stands above is pressed below, what stands below is raised on high. When there is too much, something is taken; when there is too little, something is given. ' The art of health is to preserve a firm but generous harmony.

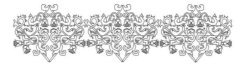

7. The Arrival of the Fatal Pulse

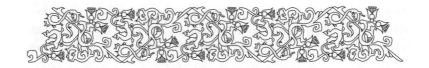

脈至浮合, 浮合如數, 一息十至以上, 是經氣予不足也. 微見九十日死.

WHEN THE PULSE ARRIVES FLOATING with its beats
joined one to the other,
Floating and joined, as if rapid, ten or more beats coming in a
single breath,
Then this is the channel qi conferring incapacity.
The pulse may be only faintly seen, but in ninety days it proves
fatal.

脈至如火薪然, 是心精之予奪也. 草乾而死.

When the pulse arrives like a fire freshly fuelled with wood,
This is the heart *jing* being stolen.
In the season when the grasses and plants wither, you die.

Li Zhongzi: Under the order of summer, fire is flourishing, and it can still add
strength and support; under the order of water (winter) the grasses dry and
wither – which means the Yang reaches its limit, which proves fatal.

脈至如散葉, 是肝氣予虛也. 木葉落而死.

When the pulse arrives like scattering leaves,
This is the liver qi conferring weakness.
When the leaves fall off the trees, you die.

脈至如省客, 省客者, 脈塞而鼓, 是腎氣予不足也. 懸去棗華而死.

When the pulse arrives like a self-effacing guest –

'A self-effacing guest' means it is blocked, sounding just like a
    drum –

This is the kidney qi conferring incapacity.

Just as the jujube bursts into blossom, you die.

Li Zhongzi: 'Scattering leaves' mean the pulse floats, drifting without a root,
and the liver qi is extremely weak. When the leaves fall off the trees, metal is
flourishing and the branches perish. Death is fitting.

Li Zhongzi: When the jujube flowers burst into blossom, earth is flourishing and
water declining, so at once it meets its end.

脈至如丸泥, 是胃精予不足也. 榆莢落而死.

When the pulse arrives faintly like a soft ball of clay,

This is the stomach *jing* conferring incapacity.

When the elm seeds are shed, you die.

脈至如橫格, 是膽氣予不足也, 禾熟而死.

When the pulse has an edge like a horizontal wooden shelf,

This is the gallbladder conferring incapacity.

As the crops ripen, so you die.

Li Zhongzi: The elm seeds are shed at the arrival of spring. At that time wood
is flourishing, and earth must be destroyed.

Li Zhongzi: The crops ripen in the autumn. Metal flourishes and wood perishes.

脈至如弦縷, 是胞精予不足也, 病善言. 下霜而死, 不言可治.

When the pulse arrives like a stretched strand of thread,

This is the heart protector's *jing* conferring incapacity.

It means you tend to talk too much.

At the fall of the frost you die – but if you cease talking it can be
    healed.

脈至如交漆, 交漆者, 左右傍至也. 微見三十日死.

When the pulse arrives as if covered by many layers of lacquer,

'Many layers of lacquer' means it is seen both left and right,

It may be hardly felt, but in thirty days you die.

Li Zhongzi: In winter months the frost falls rapidly; water arrives to overpower fire and you die. Not talking means the injury can still remain superficial, and you may be saved.

Li Zhongzi: 'Many layers of lacquer', meaning the pulse is disturbed, muddied and large. It is hardly felt when it first arrives. At the order of the moon it changes (thirty days), and the time of death arrives.

脈至如湧泉, 浮鼓肌中, 太陽氣予不足也. 少氣味. 韭英而死.

When the pulse arrives like a gushing spring, drumming
    superficially within the muscle,
This is the Taiyang qi conferring incapacity.
You feel a shortness of breath.
At the scent of onion blossoms, you die.

脈至如頹土之狀, 按之不得, 是肌氣予不足也.
五色先見黑, 白壘發死.

When the pulse arrives like the ground caving in – press down
    and it is not there –
This is the energy of the muscles conferring incapacity.
First, out of all the five colours, black is seen.
When it clearly crowds into the face, then you die.

脈至如懸雍, 懸雍者, 浮揣切之益大, 是十二俞之予不足也. 水凝而死.

When the pulse arrives as if on the brink of concord –
'On the brink of discord' means you feel for it lightly, but it
    becomes increasingly large –
It means all twelve *shu* are conferring incapacity.
When the rivers freeze over, then you die.

Li Zhongzi: When the onion blossoms come out in late summer, earth overpowers water and you die.

Li Zhongzi: Black is the colour of water. As the earth is destroyed, water turns back to 'insult' it.

Li Zhongzi: 'You feel for it lightly, but it becomes increasingly large' means having Yang without Yin, the picture of the solitary Yang rising above and becoming overbearing. The twelve 'shu' are the 'transmission' 輸 *shu* points of the *zangfu* and twelve channels. When 'the rivers freeze over', it proves fatal. The Yin qi is in abundance and the solitary Yang perishes.

脈至如偃刀, 偃刀者, 浮之小急, 按之堅大急,
五臟菀熱, 寒熱獨並於腎也, 如此其人不得坐, 立春而死.

When the pulse arrives like the back edge of a blade,

The 'back edge of a blade' means it is both superficial and slightly
tense.

Press down on it and it becomes harder and tenser.

This is the five organs having a luxuriance of heat,

Or both chills and fever coming together, solely from the kidneys.

When this happens, people are unable to sit up.

At the beginning of the spring, they die.

Li Zhongzi: To press down heavily finds the response of the kidneys...at the
order of winter, water is flourishing. It is not yet above to be destroyed. At the
meeting with spring it will prove fatal.

脈至如丸滑, 不直手, 不直手者, 按之不可得也.
是大腸氣予不足也. 棗葉生而死.

When the pulse arrives like a small slippery ball, and not straight
into the hand –

'Not coming straight into the hand' means you press on it but
cannot keep over it.

This is the large intestine qi conferring incapacity.

As the jujube leaves shoot, so they die.

脈至如華者令人善恐, 不欲坐臥, 行立常聽,
是小腸氣予不足也. 季秋而死.

When the pulse arrives like drifting flowers –

This means people tend to be fearful, but they do not want to sit
or lie down,

They walk around aimlessly, standing, and always listening –

This is the small intestine qi conferring incapacity.

At the arriving of autumn, then they die.

Li Zhongzi: The jujube leaves shoot at the start of summer. Fire is abundant
and metal perishes. Hence it proves fatal.

Li Zhongzi: The ping-fire (small intestine) declines at wu-earth. Therefore in the
season of autumn, they die.

This section evokes the manner of the fatal pulse of each organ, and the time or term of death. As each pulse falters in its own fashion, so it encounters the elements of the season – and so fails and dies. The *yinyang* and *wuxing* are used rationally here. For instance, when the pulse arrives 'like scattering leaves', which is a weakness in the liver qi (wood), then in the autumn (metal), when 'the leaves fall off the trees', you die. Metal is overpowering wood on the *wuxing* cycle. In winter (water), the grasses and plants wither, just as water conquers fire; in autumn (metal) the leaves fall off the trees, so metal conquers wood; as the jujube date blossoms during a kidney disease (water), so earth (plants and trees) conquers water; as the Chinese elm tree holds its seeds all winter but sheds them in the spring, so, with a stomach problem (earth), wood (growing things) conquers earth, and so on. This gives a rough idea of using *wuxing* science in practice. See other examples in Chapter V, Section 4, 'Further Elemental Forms and *Wuxing* Science', and Chapter IX, Sections 14–15, 'Times of Dying'.

8. The Ultimate Tool

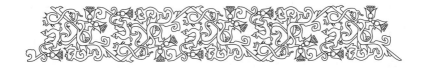

帝曰: 願聞要道. 歧伯曰:
治之要極, 無失色脈, 用之不惑, 治之大則.
逆從到行, 標本不得, 亡神失國. 去故就新, 乃得真人.

THE YELLOW EMPEROR ASKS, saying: Please, what is the key path we need to follow? Qi Bo replies:

> The ultimate task in treatment is not to neglect colour and
>   pulse.
> Make use of them, do not lose them!
> This is the great rule in treatment.
>
> When forward and backward are confused,
> When root and branch cannot be found,
> You lose the spirit – just as you would lose a country or state.
> 'Cast out the old, take on the new. '
> This is to get to the true condition in Man.

Zhang Jiebin: The key to follow when making an examination is to have a deep knowledge of pulse and colour and how their deteriorating purity comes about. Then you will not lose them. Briefly it says here if you put your hand out to a pulse *in extremis*, you may gain the kingdom. Both come together.

Zhang Jiebin: This passage here warns us in our study and advancement of virtue not to stray into the dismal world of well-worn ways, but to follow our own path of self-abandonment. 'Casting out the old' means casting off the detritus of old habits; 'taking on the new' means the work of daily advancing the new. Renewed constantly in themselves, the saints and Sages took their study to the limit, arriving at the true condition of mankind.

The most important task in treatment is not to neglect colour and pulse. To distinguish each of the characteristics of facial colour and radial pulse is to make sense of the 'ultimate tool'. With its methods you may determine the state of harmony or disharmony within. The parallels between body and state are common in classical texts. We meet this also in the next chapter, where the heart is seen as 'ruler' of the body. Zhang Jiebin's comments take these ideas to a new level, recommending daily study and practice.

9. A Common Fault
in the Pulse Exam

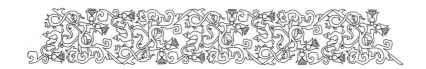

診病不問其始, 憂患飲食之失節, 起居之過度, 或傷於毒,
不先言此, 卒持寸口, 何病能中, 妄言作名, 為粗所窮.

IN DIAGNOSING A SICKNESS –

If you do not question how the sickness began,

Whether it was due to some worry or trauma, or an unrestrained
  diet or drinking,

Or whether there has been an upset to the daily routine,

Or an injury caused through some drastic medicine –

If you do not first ask about these things, but instead abruptly
  grasp hold of the 'inch-wide' mouth,

Muttering something about a sickness which can possibly have
  attacked them,

And then speak out a few vain words and give it a name –

This is 'rough treatment', given to a condition which should be
  thoroughly investigated.

The 'inch-wide' mouth is the region of the radial pulse. This
passage is repeated in Chapter VII, Section 8, with an alternative
translation. A timely warning indeed! Common faults to which
we are all prey include: not completing a history, not searching for
concomitant causes (emotional or traumatic), not identifying diet
or work stressors, not considering lifestyle, or imbalances caused

by previous interventions. Being too busy to take these into account does not befit a physician, and will render the treatment ineffective and probably worthless. Xue Shengbai comments on the profundity of pulse diagnosis:

> The pulse is the ongoing sign of qi and blood. Sickness appears in myriad forms but all we use is three fingers to fathom its transformations. If this were not the ultimate skill in the world, how could we do it? Xu Shuwei has said: 'The idea of the pulse is dark and difficult. What my heart understands, my mouth can never proclaim. ' One may use brush and ink to confer what mouth and ear impart, but these are simply rough tracings. However, despite this, if we are never acquainted with the rough, how do we sift out the smooth? Separate the pulses out, and describe them by the twenty-four pulse qualities. Do you object to there being so few? In straightened circumstances you will return to them – 'floating', 'sinking', 'tardy', 'rapid' – already you grasp the bond between them. He who attends to the pulse without distinguishing Yin and Yang will become even more tangled in his thinking!

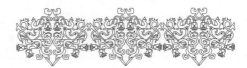

Questions for Review of Chapter IV

Indicates a more challenging question

1. Describe how to go about the examination of the pulse.

2. Explain *in your own words* how 'contrast and combine' are used in an examination. You can use looking at the pulse as an example. *

3. How does the pulse alter during the seasons? Describe its position, attachment to an organ, and character in health, in sickness and at times of fatality. Draw on your own experience if needed.

Characters in Chapter IV

pulse, vessel 脈 *mai*
contrast and combine 參伍 *canwu*
'transmission' points 輸 *shu*

V

The *Zangfu* and *Wuxing*

Through the imagery of the *zangfu* we may grasp their
inner workings and delineate a path towards health.

Key Ideas

1. *The Offices of the Zangfu*
   mutual agreement, longevity, interaction, injury, non-
   communication

2. *The Zang and their Associations*
   origins, commands, flowering, filling, taste, colour, season,
   the role of the gallbladder

3. *Directions and Elemental Associations*
   direction, entering, opening, storing, sickness, taste, class,
   beast, grain, planet, tone, number, odour

4. *Further Elemental Forms and Wuxing Science*
   direction, generation, situation in nature, voice, affect,
   bodily orifice, taste, prevailing emotion, injury, dietary
   therapy

5. *The Faculties of the Self, and their Injuries*
   human faculties, 'causal' links, injuries to the *zang*,
   diagnosis, timing death

6. *Physical Functions in Life and Death*
   the spirit before all, qi, *jin* juices, fluids, blood, vessels, the *sanjiao*, damage, the first signs of sickness

Some questions for review can be found at the end of this chapter.

1. The Offices of the *Zangfu*

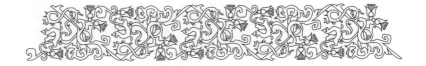

心者, 君主之官也, 神明出焉, 肺者, 相傅之官, 治節出焉.

肝者, 將軍之官, 謀慮出焉, 膽者中正之官, 決斷出焉.

膻中者, 臣使之官, 喜樂出焉, 脾胃者, 食廩之官, 五味出焉.

大腸者, 傳道之官, 變化出焉, 小腸者, 受盛之官, 化物出焉.

THE HEART IS THE OFFICE OF THE LORD and master:
A clear mind is his duty.
The lungs are the officials of communications:
Government and regulation are their duty.
The liver is the official of the military commander:
Plotting and planning are his duty.
The gallbladder is the official of inner integrity:
Making decisions and judgements are his duty.
The 'middle of the chest' is the office of the messengers:
Joy and pleasure are their duty.
The spleen and stomach are the officials of the granaries:
All foodstuffs are their duty.
The large intestines are the officials of conveyances:
Change and transformation are their duty.
The small intestines are the officials in charge of 'receiving
     fullness':
The transformation of materials is their duty.

Li Zhongzi: The small intestines reside beneath the stomach and receive the full
stomach's food and drink, separating out the pure and impure.

腎者, 作強之官, 伎巧出焉. 三焦者, 決瀆之官, 水道出焉.

膀胱者, 州都之官, 津液 藏 焉, 氣化則能出矣.

The kidneys are the officers in charge of creating vigour:

Ingenuity and skill are their duty.

The *sanjiao* is the official in charge of clearing out drains and
    waterways:

The passage of fluids is his duty.

The bladder is the office of the regional capitals:

Fluids and juices are stored therein.

The qi modifies them – so they can find a way out.

凡此十二官者, 不得相失也. 故主明則下安.

以此養生則壽. 沒世不殆, 以為天下則大昌.

Therefore, all in all, there are twelve officials,

If they cannot agree with each other, they are lost.

And so it follows:

When a master is clear-sighted, those beneath him are safe.

Use this notion in caring for life and you live long.

You are never endangered, and extending this to the whole world,

There comes an age of great brilliance!

主不明則十二官危. 使道閉塞而不通, 形乃大傷.

以此養生則殃, 以為天下者, 其宗大危, 戒之戒之.

But when the master is not clear-sighted, the twelve ministries are
    in peril.

It causes all pathways to be blocked and without communication,

And the body may then become greatly injured.

Use this plan in caring for life and there comes disaster.

Extend this to the whole world and it brings turmoil.

Beware, beware!

At the end of *Suwen* 8, in the chapter entitled 'A Secret Codex
Compiled from His Most Magical Writings', it is told how the
Yellow Emperor chose a fortunate day and hour, both deemed
lucky, to take the 'most magical writings' contained in this section,
and put them in a room specially assigned for safe-keeping, in

order to protect them for future generations. The few lines above actually comprise more than half of this valuable chapter. A 'secret codex' implies a valued collection of scrolls, or bamboo strips. In such ways the teachings of the *Neijing* were preserved. From the opening line, 'The heart is the office of the lord and master', we understand this is special territory. Each 'official' or 'office' 官 *guan* is assigned a ministry in the human frame, along with a characteristic power or emanation. Note that it is only their eventual cooperation under a 'clear-sighted' 明 *ming* ruler that creates the brilliance of the kingdom. If they cannot agree amongst themselves, they are lost.

MINISTRIES OF THE *ZANGFU*

organ	office and ministry	involvement and duties
heart	lord and master	a clear mind
lungs	communication	government and regulation
liver	military commander	plotting and planning
gallbladder	inner integrity	decisions and judgements
middle of chest	messengers	joy and pleasure
spleen and stomach	granaries	all foodstuffs
large intestines	conveyances	change and transformation
small intestines	receiving fullness	transformation of materials
kidneys	creating vigour	ingenuity and skill
sanjiao	drains and waterways	passage of all fluids
bladder	the regional capitals	storing fluids and juices

2. The *Zang* and their Associations

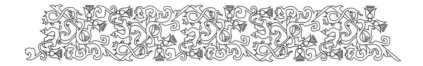

心者生之本, 神之變也, 其華在面, 其充在血脈,
為陽中之太陽, 通於夏氣.
肺者氣之本, 魄之處也, 其華在毛, 其充在皮,
為陽中之太陰, 通於秋氣.

THE HEART IS THE ORIGIN OF LIFE and transformation of
the spirit,
It flowers at the face and fills up the vessels.
It is the Taiyang in the Yang and one with the qi of the summer.
The lungs are the origin of the qi and location of the *po* soul,
They flower at the body hair and fill up the skin.
They are the Taiyin in the Yang and one with the qi of the
autumn.

腎者主蟄, 封藏之本, 精之處也, 其華在髮, 其充在骨,
為陰中之少陰, 通於冬氣.
肝者罷極之本, 魂之居也, 其華在爪, 其充在筋, 以生血氣, 其味酸,
其色蒼, 此為陽中之少陽, 通於春氣.

The kidneys are in command of hibernation and root of secure
storage,
They are the location of the purest *jing*.
They flower at the hair on the head and fill up the bones.
They are the Shaoyin in the Yin and one with the qi of
wintertime.

The liver is the origin of extreme fatigue and abode of the *hun*
   soul,
It flowers in the nails and fills up the sinews, thus producing good
   blood and qi.
Its taste is sour, its colour hoary-green.
It is the Shaoyang in the Yang and one with the qi of springtime.

脾胃大腸小腸三焦膀胱者, 食廩之本, 營之居也.
名曰器, 能化糟粕, 轉味而入出者也.
其華在唇四白, 其充在肌, 其味甘, 其色黃, 此至陰之類, 通於土氣.
凡十一臟, 取決於膽也.
The spleen and stomach, large and small intestines,
Sanjiao and bladder are the original granary halls and the abodes
   of the nutrients.
They are popularly called 'utensils' – as they are able to transform
   and move on the dregs and sediment,
Turning over the food which enters in and then passing it out.
They flower at the 'four whites' by the lips;
They fill up the muscles;
Their foodstuffs are sweet; their colour is yellow.
They are of the Ultimate Yin and one with the qi of the soil.
All the eleven organs make their decisions through the
   gallbladder.

The section beginning 'The heart is the origin of life' outlines
the individual characters of the *zangfu* and their capabilities and
associations. They are classified as 'eleven organs' (five *zang* and
six *fu*), as the ideas around the 'middle of the chest' and Heart
Protector Hand Jueyin had not crystallised at this early stage. This
chapter explains their relation in terms of Yin and Yang; their
unity with each season; and their flowering, filling and faculty. It
illustrates each of their characters – contrasting *zang* 臟 'treasury'
and *fu* 腑 'workshop' organs. In this passage, the spleen, stomach,
intestines, *sanjiao* and bladder are all named as the Ultimate Yin
(meaning 'below'). There is a rather cursory reference to the role
of the gallbladder.

TRADITIONAL CORRESPONDENCES OF THE *ZANGFU*

organs	root origin	abode	flower at	fills up	Yin and Yang	one with
heart	life	spirit	face	vessels	Taiyang in the Yang	the summer
lungs	the qi	the *po* soul	body hair	skin	Taiyin in the Yang	the autumn
kidneys	secure storage	the *jing*	head hair	bones	Shaoyin in the Yin	the winter
liver	extreme fatigue	the *hun* soul	nails	sinews	Shaoyang in the Yang	the spring
spleen, stomach, intestines	granary halls	nutrients	'four whites' by the lips	muscles	Ultimate Yin	the soil
gallbladder	all eleven organs make their decisions through the gallbladder					

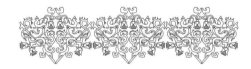

3. Directions and Elemental Associations

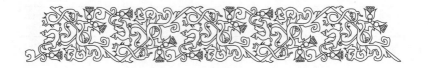

東方青色, 入通於肝, 開竅於目, 藏精於肝. 其病發驚駭.

其味酸, 其類草木, 其畜雞, 其穀麥.

其應四時, 上為歲星, 是以春氣在頭也.

其音角, 其數八, 是以知病之在筋也. 其臭臊.

THE EASTERLY DIRECTION: ITS COLOUR IS BLUE-
   GREEN.

It enters into the liver, opens out into the eyes and stores its *jing*
   in the liver.

Its sickness develops through being frightened or shocked.

Its taste is sour; it is classed with vegetation and trees, its beast is
   the cockerel, its grain is wheat.

In response to the seasons it occupies the planet Jupiter above.

Therefore in the springtime its qi is present in the head.

Its tone is '*jue*'; its number eight.

It causes you to perceive its sickness in the sinews; its odour is
   rank.

南方赤色, 入通於心, 開竅於耳, 藏於心, 故病在五臟.

其味苦, 其類火, 其畜羊, 其穀黍.

其應四時, 上為熒惑星. 是以知病之在脈也.

其音征, 其數七, 其臭焦.

The southerly direction: its colour is red.

It enters into the heart, opens out into the ears and stores its *jing*
   in the heart.

156

Thus its sickness is present in all five *zang*.

Its taste is bitter; it is classed with 'fire', its beast is the goat, its grain is millet.

In response to the seasons it occupies the fiery planet Mars above.

It causes you to perceive its sickness in the vessels.

Its tone is '*zhi*'; its number seven; its odour is scorched.

中央黃色, 入通於脾, 開竅於口, 藏精於脾, 故病在舌本.
其味甘, 其類土, 其畜牛, 其穀稷.
其應四時, 上為鎮星. 是以知病之在肉也.
其音宮, 其數五, 其臭香.

The 'central region': its colour is yellow.

It enters into the spleen, opens out into the mouth and stores its *jing* in the spleen.

Thus its sickness lies at the root of the tongue.

Its taste is sweet; it is classed with 'soil', its beast is the ox,

Its grain is panicled millet.

In response to the seasons it occupies the planet Saturn above.

It causes you to perceive its sickness in the flesh.

Its tone is '*gong*'; its number five; its odour is fragrant.

西方白色, 入通於肺, 開竅於鼻, 藏精於肺, 故病背.
其味辛, 其類金, 其畜馬, 其穀稻.
其應四時, 上為太白星. 是以知病之在皮毛也.
其音商, 其數九, 其臭腥.

The westerly region: its colour is white.

It enters into the lungs; it opens out into the nostrils

And stores its *jing* in the lungs, causing its sickness to be present in the back.

Its taste is pungent; it is classed with 'metals', its beast is the horse, its grain is rice grown in flooded fields.

In response to the seasons it occupies the pale star Venus above.

It causes you to perceive its sickness in the skin and hair.

Its tone is '*shang*', its number nine, its odour is rotten.

北方黑色, 入通於腎, 開竅於二陰, 藏精於腎, 故病在谿.

其味鹹, 其類水, 其畜彘, 其穀豆.

其應四時, 上為辰星. 是以知病之在骨也.

其音羽, 其數六, 其臭腐.

The northerly direction: its colour is black.

It enters into the kidneys; it opens out into the two 'lower
     openings' and stores its *jing* in the kidneys,

Causing its sickness to be present in the 'streams' between the
     muscles.

Its taste is salty; it is classed with 'water', its animal is the swine,
     its grain is peas and beans.

In response to the seasons it occupies the planet Mercury above.

It causes you to perceive its sickness in the bones.

Its tone is '*yu*'; its number six; its odour is stale.

These lines are often quoted; indeed they are the *locus classicus*
of the many and varied *wuxing* associations. There is no more
important text for traditional Chinese science. It shows the
sweeping brief of the Warring States and Han natural thinking;
and clearly illustrates an associative logic – in contradistinction to
the more formal atomism of the Greeks. The almost ceremonial
recitation of the five elements and their associations illustrates
meticulously the concrete logic of 'mysterious mutual mixing'.
Five cardinal directions are mentioned – east, west, central,
south, north (including central) – but the text gives precedence
to geography, as it develops its very own meta-logic (or eco-logic)
of the natural world. The *direction* is listed first, to identify *place*
(east first, where the sun rises), then colour, and then how colour
(elemental qi/energy vibration) enters into each organ; then
corresponding opening and origin, organ, sense and characteristic
sickness. Then comes responding taste, elemental class, beast and
grain, planet, number, particular tissue, tone and odour. The tones
correspond to the five notes of the pentatonic scale. The whole has
the flavour of the shamanic gloss or rubric, a ritual prayer to the
spirit of Gaia.

4. Further Elemental Forms and *Wuxing* Science

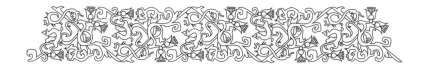

東方生風, 風生木, 木生酸, 酸生肝, 肝生筋, 筋生心.
肝主目, 其在天為玄, 在人為道, 在地為化.
化生五味, 道生智, 玄生神, 神在天為風.
在地為木, 在體為筋, 在臟為肝. 在色為蒼, 在音為角, 在聲為呼,
在變動為握, 在竅為目, 在味為酸, 在志為怒. 怒傷肝, 悲勝怒.
風傷筋, 燥勝風, 酸傷筋, 辛勝酸.

THE EASTERLY DIRECTION GENERATES WIND; wind generates wood; wood generates sourness; sourness generates the liver; the liver generates the sinews; the sinews generate the heart.

> The liver is in command of the eyes.
> In respect of the skies it creates darkness,
> In respect of man it forms the Way.
> On earth it appears as transformations.
> In transforming it generates the 'five tastes',
> As the Way it generates wisdom.
> As darkness it generates the spirit.
> As the spirit in the skies it makes for the wind.

On the earth it appears in the trees; in the body it is the sinews; among organs it is the liver; among colours it is hoary green; among notes it is '*jue*'; among voices it is those shouting; on being affected it creates spasms; among openings it is the eyes; among tastes it is those sour; among emotions it represents anger.

> Anger injures the liver,
> Grief prevails over anger.

The wind injures the sinews; dryness prevails over the wind. Sour tastes injure the sinews; the pungent prevails over the sour.

南方生熱, 熱生火, 火生苦, 苦生心, 心生血, 血生脾.
心主舌, 其在天為熱, 在地為火.
在體為脈, 在臟為心, 在色為赤, 在音為徵, 在聲為笑,
在變動為憂, 在竅為舌, 在味為苦, 在志為喜. 喜傷心, 恐勝喜.
熱傷氣, 寒勝熱. 苦傷氣, 鹹勝苦.

The southerly direction generates heat; heat generates fire; fire generates bitterness; bitterness generates the heart; the heart generates blood; blood generates the spleen.

> The heart is in command of the tongue.
> In the skies it appears as heat,
> On earth it becomes flames and fire.

In the body it appears as the blood-pulse; among organs it is the heart; among colours it is the red; among tones it is 'zhi'; among voices it is those laughing; on being affected it creates sadness; among openings it is the tongue; among tastes it is those bitter; among emotions it represents joy.

> Joy injures the heart,
> Fear prevails over joy.

Heat injures qi; cold prevails over heat. Bitter tastes injure the qi; salty prevails over bitter.

中央生濕, 濕生土, 土生甘, 甘生脾, 脾生肉, 肉生肺.
脾主口, 其在天為濕, 在地為土.
在體為肉, 在臟為脾, 在色為黃, 在音為宮, 在聲為歌,
在變動為噦, 在竅為口, 在味為甘, 在志為思. 思傷脾, 怒勝思.
濕傷肉, 風勝濕, 甘傷肉, 酸勝甘.

The central region generates damp; dampness generates the soil; the soil generates sweetness; sweetness generates the spleen; the spleen generates the flesh; the flesh generates the lungs.

The spleen is in command of the mouth.
In the skies it appears as dampness,
On the earth it appears in the soil.

In the body it is the flesh; among organs it is the spleen; among colours it is yellow; among tones it is '*gong*'; among voices it is those singing; on being affected it means breaking wind; among openings it is the mouth; among tastes it is those sweet; among emotions it represents deliberation.

Deliberation injures the spleen,
Anger prevails over deliberation.

Dampness injures flesh; the wind prevails over dampness. Sweet tastes injure the flesh; sour prevails over sweet.

西方生燥, 燥生金, 金生辛, 辛生肺, 肺生皮毛, 皮毛在腎.
肺主鼻, 其在天為燥, 在地為金.
在體為皮毛, 在臟為肺, 在色為白, 在音為商, 在聲為哭,
在變動為咳, 在竅為鼻, 在味為辛, 在志為憂. 憂傷肺, 喜勝憂.
熱傷皮毛, 寒勝熱, 辛傷皮毛, 苦勝辛.

The westerly direction generates dryness; dryness generates metal; metal generates pungency; pungency generates the lungs; the lungs generate the skin and hair; the skin and hair generate the kidneys.

The lungs are in command of the nostrils.
In the skies it appears as dryness,
On the earth it represents in metals.

In the body it is the skin and hair; among organs it is the lungs; among colours it is white; among tones it is '*shang*'; among voices it is those weeping; on being affected it creates coughing; among openings it is the nostrils; among tastes it is those pungent; among emotions it represents sadness.

Sadness injures the lungs,
Joy prevails over sadness.

The heat injures the skin and hair; cold prevails over heat. Pungent tastes injure the skin and hair; bitter prevails over pungent.

北方生寒, 寒生水, 水生鹹, 鹹生腎, 腎生骨髓, 髓生肝.
腎主耳, 其在天為寒, 在地為水.
在體為骨, 在臟為腎, 在色為黑, 在音為羽, 在聲為呻,
在變動為慄, 在竅為耳, 在味為鹹, 在志為恐. 恐傷腎, 思勝恐.
寒傷血, 燥勝寒, 鹹傷血, 甘勝鹹.

The northerly direction generates cold; cold generates water; water generates saltiness; saltiness generates the kidneys; the kidneys generate the bones and marrow; the marrow generates the liver.

> The kidneys are in command of the ears.
> In the skies it appears as coldness,
> On the earth it becomes water.

In the body it is in the bones; among organs it is the kidneys; among colours it means blackness; among tones it is '*yu*'; among voices it is those groaning; on being affected it creates trembling; among openings it is the ears; among tastes is those salty; among emotions it represents fear.

> Fear injures the kidneys,
> Deliberation prevails over fear.

The cold injures the blood; dryness prevails over cold. Salty tastes injure the blood; sweet prevails over salty.

Another ritual gloss from the Warring States and Han. For a second time, the five directions are listed (east, south, central, west, north) with their corresponding powers and elements. Again note the cardinal importance of direction, or *place*. The text shows the first stirrings of geomancy or *feng shui* ('wind-water'), before it developed into an extended school. The people of pre-Han times had an acute sensitivity to place, and a concrete perception of their natural environment, as shown in the listings. These include their inner attributes: the sound of the voice, the effect on the body, a preferential taste and emotion. 'The easterly direction generates wind; wind generates wood; wood generates sourness; sourness generates the liver...' – the entire passage shows the morphogenesis of the individual. It is as if our very being came 'from nature', a blending of the forces surrounding us with no need for a first cause or paternal (that is, Judaic) creator. Certainly such a view borders on the realm of 'gods and spirits' 神鬼 *shengui*, but this is commonplace in early medicine. Medicine and sorcery have often been uneasy bedfellows.

The great significance of these last two selections is that they reveal a panoply of *wuxing* science, a complete range of directional and elemental associations. The texts show how the *yinyang* and *wuxing* work ultimately through encouragement and restraint – a resonance and dissonance, between elements. They show a tapestry of causal accident, known by Chinese science as the registries of 'mutual generation' 相生 *xiangsheng*, wood produces fire, fire produces earth (ashes), earth yields metals, and so on, and 'mutual control' 相克 *xiangke*, earth controls water (as in a dam), water controls fire, fire controls metal (as in smelting), and so on. Our modern imagination may just be the 'poor cousin' to the much richer world of the primitive. The eidetic memory and awareness possessed by these peoples, immersed in the womb of nature, was critical in producing a psychology of associative thinking.

Each string of associations ends with identifying an opening, a taste, a voice – shouting, laughing, singing, weeping, groaning – and an associated emotion. It was understood very early on that emotions, unchecked, could damage health – while conversely the expression of an emotion could heal. This view, rather remarkably, foreshadows psychotherapy by some 2000 years. Emotion means a sounding-out, resonance or echo of the 'sound' of the natural world: wood (growing things, 'bursting') reveals outgoing aggression and anger, fire (flowering and 'blooming') makes for joy, metal ('settling', dry and cold) comes as grief, while water (unstable, powerful, 'storing') completely populates us, creating hesitation and fear, and so on. These emotions are a further expression of the cycle of spring, summer, autumn and winter: the 'birth and growth, closure and storage' 生長, 收藏 *shengzhang, shouzang* beat which makes up the year:

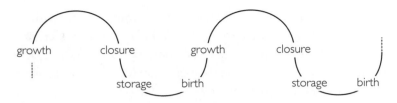

– summer – autumn – winter – spring – summer – autumn – winter – spring –

Birth and growth, closure and storage

Here the *yinyang* is at work, both in the person (small heaven) and in the wide world (large Heaven). I believe it shows four things about ourselves:

1. We are one with nature, we cannot be separated out from it.

2. That emotions are the binding force between us and the world.

3. Balance and order can be established through an emotional life.

4. Finally, balance may be re-established by finding the controlling emotion.

What is asserted is that we are one body physically with our immediate surroundings – both a blunt sensory awareness, and a fine, barely felt perception of a looming world. As Laozi says: 'Watch…it cannot be seen; listen…it cannot be heard; grasp… it cannot be held. ' Our feelings bind us to the concrete. But, more important, balance or health may be re-established by one emotion regulating or controlling another. Mencius says it is the feelings of compassion, shame and humility, and our innate sense of right and wrong, that make us human-hearted. These are the beginning of true wisdom. I believe this explains the popularity of relaxation skills, complementary therapies, meditation practices, mindfulness and psychotherapy. Hormonal equilibrium is re-established by allowing all agencies of the body mutual recognition, subsequent validation, and consequently the self-regulation of the *yinyang*.

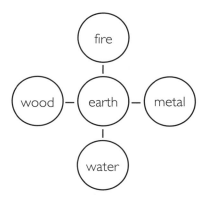

A basic *wuxing* diagram

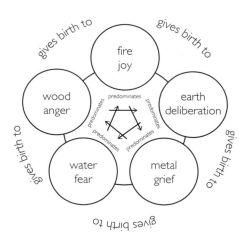

A complete *wuxing* diagram of the governance of the emotions

PENTATONIC TONE, ELEMENT AND ASPECT

	pentatonic soh fire – 征 *zhi* south	
pentatonic mi wood – 角 *jue* east	pentatonic doh soil – 宮 *gong* central	pentatonic ray metal – 商 *shang* west
	pentatonic lah water – 羽 *yu* north	

FIVE DIRECTIONS WITH
TRADITIONAL ASSOCIATIONS

easterly	southerly	central	westerly	northerly
blue-green	red	yellow	white	black
enters into liver	enters into heart	enters into spleen	enters into lungs	enters into kidneys
opens into eyes	opens into ears	opens into mouth	opens into nostrils	opens below
essences in liver	essences in heart	essences in spleen	essences in lungs	essences in kidneys
sickness through being frightened or shocked	sickness lies in all five *zang* organs	sickness lies at the root of the tongue	sickness presents in the back	sickness in 'streams' between the muscles
sour	bitter	sweet	pungent	salty
vegetation and trees	fire	soil	metals	water
the cockerel	the goat	the ox	the horse	the swine
wheat	millet	panicled millet	rice in flooded fields	peas and beans
the planet Jupiter	the planet Mars	the planet Saturn	the planet Venus	the planet Mercury
sickness in sinews	sickness in vessels	sickness in flesh	sickness in skin or hair	sickness in bones
the tone *jue*	the tone *zhi*	the tone *gong*	the tone *shang*	the tone *yu*
8	7	5	9	6
a rank odour	a scorched odour	a fragrant odour	a rotten odour	a stale odour

5. The Faculties of the Self, and their Injuries

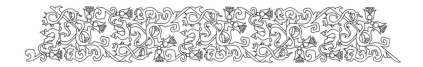

天之在我者德也, 地之在我者氣也. 德流氣薄而生者也.
故生之來謂之精, 兩精相搏謂之神.

THE SKIES ARE PRESENT WITHIN THE SELF as virtue,
The land is present within the self as qi.
Virtue streams forth and the breath thins out –
And thus is brought about human life.
Thereafter life is brought about due to the *jing*,
And both *jing* are drawn together as 'spirit'.

隨神往來者謂之魂, 並精而出入者謂之魄,
所以任物者謂之心, 心有所憶謂之意, 意之所存謂之志.

It follows the spirit in its arrival and departure –
This is known as the '*hun* soul'.
It accompanies the essences as they exit and enter –
This is known as the '*po* soul'.
It bears responsibility for all things –
This is known as the 'heart'.
That which is reflected upon in the heart –
This constitutes the 'mind'.
That which is kept in the mind –
This constitutes the 'will'.

因志而存變謂之思, 因思而遠慕謂之慮, 因慮而處物謂之智.

Because of the will guarding against change, we have 'thinking'.

Because of thinking and far-off longing, we have 'worrying'.

Because of worrying and trying to manage things, we come to
    what is called 'wisdom'.

心怵惕思慮則傷神, 神傷則恐懼自失.

破䐃脫肉, 毛悴色夭死於冬.

Once the heart becomes apprehensive,

You start thinking and worrying, which injures the spirit.

If you injure the spirit, you become frightened

And over-cautious about your own preservation.

It tears your body shape and you lose weight,

The body hair becomes bedraggled,

The face dries out, and it brings death in the winter.

脾愁憂而不解則傷意, 意傷則悗亂.

四肢不舉, 毛悴色夭死於春.

Once the spleen becomes downcast

And depressed, with no let-up, it injures the mind.

If it injures the mind, you hang your head,

As if bowed down by catastrophe.

The four limbs will not lift up,

The body hair becomes bedraggled,

The face dries out, and it brings death in the spring.

肝悲哀動中則傷魂, 魂傷則狂忘不精.

不精則不正, 當人陰縮而攣筋, 兩脅骨不舉, 毛悴色夭死於秋.

Once the liver becomes griefstricken,

As sobbing stirs within, it injures the *hun* soul.

If it injures the *hun* soul, it produces incoherent behaviour,

Disorientation and lack of clarity.

With lack of clarity, your behaviour becomes improper.

It makes a man's sex organ retract and contracts his sinews.

The sides of the ribcage cannot be raised up,

The body hair becomes bedraggled,

The face dries out, and it brings death in the autumn.

肺喜樂無極則傷魄, 魄傷則狂,

狂者意不存人, 皮革焦, 毛悴色夭死於夏.

Once the lungs feel joy and pleasure without limit,

It injures the *po* soul.

If you injure the *po* soul, it produces incoherent behaviour.

Incoherent behaviour means you think of no one but yourself,

Your skin turns leathery and becomes heated;

The body hair becomes bedraggled,

The face dries out, and it brings death in the summer.

腎盛怒而不止則傷志, 志傷則喜忘其前言,

腰脊不可以俛仰屈伸, 毛悴色夭死於季夏.

Once the kidneys are full of an anger which is relentless,

It injures the will.

If it injures the will, you tend to forget what has just been
　　remarked upon.

The waist and spine cannot bend forward or back, stretch either
　　up or down.

The body hair becomes bedraggled,

The face dries out and it brings death in the late summer.

恐懼而不解則傷精, 精傷則骨痠痿厥, 精時自下.

Once you become fearful and overcautious, with no let-up, it
　　injures the *jing*.

If you injure the *jing*, the bones will wither and weaken,

And the *jing* itself, in time, decreases.

A precious text. The section beginning 'The skies are present
within the self as virtue', in clear and unequivocal fashion, defines
the creation of virtue, the qi, human life, *jing*, the spirit, *hun* 魂
and *po* 魄 soul, the will, thought, worrying and wisdom as they
occur within the human frame – and also how they interlink. The
text considers the origins of human life and the occurrence of each
mental strength. A symptomology is developed for the breakdown
of the five *zang*. The heart may become over-fearful, the spleen
distressed, the liver griefstricken, the lungs over-pleasured, and the
kidneys full of anger. Excess emotion leads to an injury to physical
health, which occurs at a particular season.

6. Physical Functions in Life and Death

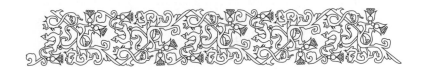

黃帝曰: 余聞人有精, 氣, 津, 液, 血, 脈, 余意以為一氣耳,
今乃辨為六名, 余不知其所以然.

THE YELLOW EMPEROR ASKS: I have heard that:
All people have *jing*, qi, fluids, juices, blood and blood vessels.
I understand they are merely one qi.
Now we divide them up to have six different names.
I do not understand why we do this.

岐伯曰: 兩神相搏, 合而成形.
常先身生, 是謂精.

Qi Bo replies: As both fine spirits are drawn to each other,
They fit into each other to complete the human frame.
This always precedes the life of the physical body. It is the
  function of the *jing*.

何謂氣? 上焦開發, 宣五谷味. 熏膚, 充身, 澤毛.
若霧露之溉, 是謂氣.

And what about the qi?
The upper *jiao* opens up, spreading out wide the flavours of the
  five grains.
They send their vapours up into the skin, filling the body and
  moistening its body hair.
It is like being soaked through by a damp mist or dew.
This is the function of the qi.

何謂津? 腠理發泄, 汗出溱溱, 是謂津.

And what about the 'juices'?

The pores of the skin express outwardly and dissipate, and sweat appears throughout.

This is the function of the 'juices'.

何謂液? 穀入氣滿, 淖澤注於骨.

骨屬屈伸, 泄澤補益腦髓, 皮膚潤澤, 是謂液.

And what about the 'fluids'?

When food is taken in, the *qi* becomes filled.

It oozes and gently seeps into the bones.

The bones by nature are for bending and stretching.

They then disperse it out further to moisten and benefit the brain and bone marrow, and the skin is enriched and glistens.

This is the function of the 'fluids'.

何謂血? 中焦受氣, 取汁變化而赤, 是謂血.

And what about the 'blood'?

As the middle *jiao* receives the qi, it gets a juice which is changed and transforms, turning red.

This makes for the 'blood'.

何謂脈? 壅遏營氣, 令無所避, 是謂脈.

And what about the 'vessels'?

Stopping and preventing the nutrient qi leaking away and making sure none escapes.

This is the function of the 'vessels'.

精脫者, 耳聾, 氣脫者, 目不明, 津脫者, 腠理開, 汗大泄.

液脫者, 骨屬屈伸不利, 色夭, 腦髓消, 脛痠, 耳數鳴.

血脫者, 色白, 夭然不澤.

When the *jing* is squandered, the ears become deaf.

When the qi is squandered, the eyes become unclear.

When the juices are squandered, the texture of the skin opens out and the sweat greatly dissipates.

When the fluids are squandered, the bones, normally used for bending and stretching, can no longer be used.

The face dries out, the brain and bone marrow shrink,
The calves ache and the ears hear a constant sound.
As the blood is squandered, the face turns pale, dries out and no
    longer glistens clear.

The passage beginning 'As both fine spirits are drawn to each other' yields a picture of how life comes together in the womb. As Yin and Yang *hun* and *po* spirits are drawn in close proximity to one another, human life comes into being. What follows is a clear view of how various substances also come into existence and their function in the body, with particular reference to the *sanjiao*. The *jing*, qi, *jin* juices, fluids, blood and vessels are listed. The final verse outlines the signs of sickness upon the loss of each. In Li Zhongzi's original work the whole of this chapter was entitled 'Zang Imagery' 臟象 *zangxiang*, perhaps implying a description of the 'images and shapes of the *zang* organs'. But the character *zang* can mean 'hidden' and *xiang* can mean 'revealed'. Thus it is in the nature of the organs to be, at one time, both somewhat obvious and somewhat hidden. Through their imagery we grasp their inner workings and may delineate a path towards health. Here is Xue Shengbai's comment:

That which divides the *zang* from the *fu* is something almost too small to be seen – it really is minute and infinitesimal. But to point us in the right direction we have this chapter on the 'images and shapes of the *zang* organs'. Once the ancients had arrived at a spiritual understanding of things, it was as if they were seeing through a wall with its other side illuminated. They used this method, and this method alone. But change and transformation are never-ending, never-ceasing – it is impossible to take anything as a fixed rule – all we have are images and shapes, and it is true that it is images and shapes alone which are spiritual! It is said: 'Abandon the image and you grope in the dark. ' So stick to what you can see, and await the hare!

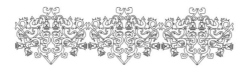

Questions for Review of Chapter V
* Indicates a more challenging question

1. List the main offices and duties in the body of the heart, lungs, liver, gallbladder, 'middle of the chest', spleen and stomach, large and small intestines, kidneys, *sanjiao* and bladder.

2. Expand on the saying: 'When the master is not clear-sighted, the twelve ministries are in peril.'*

3. Draw a table to illustrate the associations and characters of the four organs: heart, lungs, kidneys and liver.

4. Draw a table to show how direction is linked to colour, organ, opening, storing, developing sickness, taste, class, beast, grain, planet, perceived sickness, tone, number and odour.

5. How do emotions correspond to elemental forces, especially with reference to *wuxing* science? Explain why their interactions can cause disease. Use a diagram.

6. Do you think that diet can influence emotion and cause disease? Expand on your views. *

Characters in Chapter V

CHINESE EXTRACTS

heart 心 *xin*

lungs 肺 *fei*

liver 肝 *gan*

gallbladder 膽 *dan*

'middle of chest' 膻中 *sanzhong*

spleen 脾 *pi*

stomach 胃 *wei*

large intestines 大腸 *da chang*

small intestines 小腸 *xian chang*

kidneys 腎 *shen*

sanjiao 三焦 *sanjiao*

bladder 膀胱 *pangguang*

GENERAL TEXT

official, office 官 *guan*

clear-sighted, enlightened 明 *ming*

solid, 'treasury' organ 臟 *zang*

more hollow, 'workshop' organ 腑 *fu*

mutual generation (wood produces fire, fire produces earth (ashes), earth yields metals, and so on) 相生 *xiangsheng*

mutual control (earth dams water, water dowses fire, fire smelts metals, and so on) 相克 *xiangke*

birth and growth, closure and storage 生長, 收藏 *shengzhang, shouzang*

***hun* soul** 魂 *hun*

***po* soul** 魄 *po*

***zang* imagery** (suggesting the *zang* organs) 臟象 *zangxiang*

VI

Channels and Collaterals

As the *zangfu* are the roots of the Jingluo, so the
Jingluo represent their stalks and leaves.

Key Ideas

1. *The Form and Length of the Channels*
   the twelve Jingluo, Lungs hand Taiyin, Large Intestine hand
   Yangming, Stomach foot Yangming, Spleen foot Taiyin,
   Heart hand Shaoyin, Small Intestine hand Taiyang, Bladder
   foot Taiyang, Kidney foot Shaoyin, Heart lord hand Jueyin,
   Sanjiao hand Shaoyang, Gallbladder foot Shaoyang, Liver
   foot Jueyin, the Conception and Governor vessels

A question for review can be found at the end of this chapter.

1. The Form and Length of the Channels

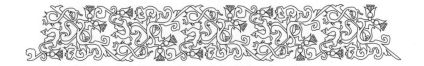

肺手太陰之脈, 起於中焦, 下絡大腸, 還循胃口, 上膈屬肺.
從肺系橫出腋下, 下循臑內行少陰心主之前下肘中,
循臂內上骨下廉入寸口, 上魚, 循魚際出大指之端.
其支者, 從腕後直出次指內廉, 出其端.

THE LUNGS HAND TAIYIN VESSEL rises at the middle *Jiao*,
And travels down to connect up with the Large Intestine,
Circles back along following the mouth of the stomach,
And travels up through the diaphragm to belong to the lungs.
From the system of the lungs it crosses over horizontally to come
    out under the armpit, and travels down
Following along the inside of the upper arm, passing in front of
    the Shaoyin and Heart lord channels,
Travels down into the elbow,
Following along the inside of the forearm,
And up past the lower edge of the bone to enter into the 'inch-
    wide mouth'.
It passes up to the 'fish' and follows along the 'border of the fish',
    to come out at the thumb's tip.

A branch, from behind the wrist, comes out directly,
Travelling along the inner edge of the next finger, coming out at
    its tip.

大腸手陽明之脈, 起於大指次指之端, 循指上廉出合谷兩骨之間.
上入兩筋之中, 循臂上廉入肘外廉, 上臑外前廉, 上肩出骨禺骨之前廉,
上出於柱骨之會上, 下入缺盆絡肺, 下膈屬大腸.
其支者, 從缺盆上頸貫頰入下齒中, 還出挾口交人中,
左之右, 右之左, 上挾鼻孔.

THE LARGE INTESTINE HAND YANGMING VESSEL rises
    at the tip of the finger next to the thumb,
Follows along the upper edge of the finger, to come out at the
    'joining valleys', between the two bones.
It travels up to enter in between the two tendons,
Follows along the upper edge of the forearm,
Enters into the outer edge of the elbow,
Follows up the outer front edge of the upper arm, up to the
    shoulder,
Coming out at the front edge, on the collar bone.
It travels on up to come out at the joining at the 'column bone',
Travelling down to enter into the 'broken basin',
Connects up with the lungs, and passes down through the
    diaphragm to belong to the Large Intestine.

A branch, from the 'broken basin', travels directly upwards over
    the neck to pass through the cheek,
Entering in below the teeth,
Circling back to come out alongside the mouth,
Crossing over at the 'middle man', left going right, right going
    left –
Then travelling upwards to besides the nostrils.

胃足陽明之脈, 起於鼻, 交頞中, 旁納太陽之脈.
下循鼻外入上齒中, 還出挾口環脣下交承漿, 卻循頤後下廉出大迎,
從頰車上耳前, 過客主人, 循際至額顱.
其支者, 從大迎前下人迎, 循喉嚨入缺盆, 下膈屬胃絡脾.
其直者, 從缺盆下乳內廉, 下挾臍入氣街中.
其支者, 起於胃口, 下循腹裡下至氣街中而合, 以下髀關, 抵伏兔,
下膝臏中, 下循脛外廉下足跗, 入中指內間.
其支者, 下廉三寸而別入中指外間. 其支者, 別跗上入大指間, 出其端.

THE STOMACH FOOT YANGMING VESSEL rises at
    the nose,

Crosses over the middle of the lower forehead,

And inserts beside it, into the vessel of the Taiyang.

Travelling down, it follows the outside of the nose, and enters
    into the top teeth.

It circles back, coming out both sides of the mouth, ringing the
    lips,

And then travelling down to intersect at 'receiving fluid'.

It follows behind to the back edge of the lower jaw, coming out at
    the 'great welcome',

Following the 'cheek carriage', travelling up in front of the ear,

To pass over the 'guest and host' and following the border of the
    hair

To arrive at the bony part at the front of the skull.

A branch, from in front of 'great welcome', travels down to
    'people welcome',

Following the windpipe to enter into the 'broken basin',

Travels down through the diaphragm to belong to the stomach
    and connect up with the Spleen.

From the 'broken basin', the vessel travels on directly down the
    inner edge of the breast,

Besides the navel, to enter into the 'qi highway'.

Another branch rises at the mouth of the stomach and follows on
    down, lining the belly,

To arrive at the 'qi highway' where they reunite.

From there it travels down through 'thigh pass', reaching
    'crouched rabbit',

Down to enter the kneecap, follows on down the outer edge of
    the shin,

Down to the instep, to enter the inner gap by the middle toe.

Another branch, from three inches under the knee,

Separates out and travels down to enter the outer gap by the
    middle toe.

Another branch separates out from above the instep,

To enter the gap by the big toe, and comes out at its tip.

脾足太陰之脈, 起於大指之端, 循指內側白肉際過核骨後, 上內踝前廉.
上踹內, 循脛骨後交出厥陰之前, 上膝股內前廉, 入腹屬脾絡胃,
上膈挾咽, 連舌本, 散舌下.
其支者, 復從胃別上膈注心中.

THE SPLEEN FOOT TAIYIN VESSEL rises at the tip of the
     big toe,
Follows along the inner surface of the toe at the border of the
     white flesh,
Passing over behind the 'walnut bone', to travel up the front edge
     of the inner ankle.
It travels up the inner calf, following along behind the shinbone,
Crossing over and coming out in front of the Jueyin,
Travels up following to the knee and inner front edge of the thigh,
And enters the belly, where it belongs to the Spleen and connects
     up with the Stomach.
It travels up to the diaphragm, beside the throat, linking up at the
     root of the tongue,
And scattering in under the tongue.

A branch, also from the Stomach, separates out and travels up to
     the diaphragm, to pour into the Heart.

心手少陰之脈, 起於心中, 出屬心系, 下膈絡小腸.
其支者, 從心系上挾咽系目系.
其直者, 復從心系卻上肺, 下出腋下,
下循臑內後廉行太陰心主之後下肘內, 循臂內後廉抵掌後銳骨之端.
入掌內後廉, 循小指之內出其端.

THE HEART HAND SHAOYIN VESSEL rises from within the
     heart, and comes out to belong to the system of the heart,
Travelling down to the diaphragm, to connect up with the Small
     Intestine.
A branch from the system of the heart travels up beside the
     throat, to tie up with the system of the eye.

Another branch, from the system of the heart, travels back to
     under the lungs to come out under the armpit.
It follows on down the inner back edge of the upper arm,

Following behind the Taiyin and Heart lord,

Travelling down into the inner edge of the elbow,

Following the inner back edge of the forearm, to reach the tip of
the 'joy bone' behind the palm.

There it enters the inner back edge of the palm, following the
inside of the little finger, to come out at its tip.

小腸手太陽之脈, 起於小指之端, 循手外側上腕, 出踝中.

直上循臂骨下廉出肘內側兩筋之間, 上循臑外後廉出肩解,

繞肩胛交肩上, 入缺盆絡心, 循咽下膈抵胃小腸.

其支者, 從缺盆循頸上頰至目銳眦上, 卻入耳中.

其支者, 別循頰上䪼抵鼻, 至目內眦, 斜絡於顴.

THE SMALL INTESTINE HAND TAIYANG VESSEL rises at
the tip of the little finger,

Following along the outer surface of the hand up to the wrist,

Coming out among the bones of the wrist.

It travels directly up, following along the lower edge of the bone
of the forearm,

To come out at the inner surface of the elbow, at the space
between the two bones.

It travels on up, following the outer back edge of the forearm, to
come out at the loosening part of the shoulder,

Entwines the shoulder blade and crosses over above the shoulder,

To enter the 'broken basin' and connect up with the Heart,

Following the throat, down to the diaphragm,

To reach the stomach and belong to the Small Intestine.

A branch, from the 'broken basin', follows up the neck to the
cheek,

Arriving at the outer corner of the eye,

And turning back enters into the ear.

Another branch separately follows up the cheek, below the eye, to
reach the nose,

Arriving at the inner corner of the eye,

Travelling slantwise across to connect up at the cheek.

膀胱足太陽之脈, 起於目內, 上額交巔.
其支者, 從巔至耳上角, 其直者, 從巔入絡腦, 還出別下項,
循肩髆內挾脊抵腰中, 入循膂絡腎屬膀胱.
其支者, 從腰中下挾脊貫臀入膕中.
其支者, 從髆內左右別下貫胛, 挾脊內過髀樞, 循髀外從後廉下合膕中,
　　以下貫踹內, 出外踝之後, 循京骨至小指外側.

THE BLADDER FOOT TAIYANG VESSEL rises at the inner
    corner of the eye,
Travelling up over the forehead to cross over at the crown.
A branch, from the crown, follows on
To arrive at the upper corner of the ear,
And directly, from the crown, enters in to connect up with the
    brain,
Circles back, comes out and separates out
To travel down the nape of the neck,
Passing by inside the shoulder blade,
Besides the spine, to reach into the waist,
And descending down either side of the backbone reaches the
    waist,
Where it enters in, following the spine to connect up with the
    Kidney and belong to the Bladder.

A branch, from within the waist, travels down either side of the
    spine,
Passing directly through the buttocks to enter into the hollow in
    the back of the knee.

Another branch, from inside the shoulder blade, left and right,
Separates out to travel down,
Passing directly through the flesh either side of the spine,
To enter in and pass over the hip joint.
It follows the outer back edge of the buttock,
Travelling down to reunite in the hollow at the back of the knee.
Thereby it travels on down directly entering the calf, to come out
Behind the outer ankle, following the 'capital bone',
To reach down clear to the outer surface of the little toe.

腎足少陰之脈, 起於小指之下, 斜走足心,
出於然谷之下, 循內踝之後別入跟中.
以上端內, 出膕內廉, 上股內後廉, 貫脊屬腎絡膀胱.
其直者, 從腎上貫肝膈入肺中, 循喉嚨挾舌本.
其支者, 從肺出絡心, 注胸中.

THE KIDNEY FOOT SHAOYIN VESSEL rises from under the
    little toe,

And runs slantwise across the sole of the foot,

Coming out under the 'blazing valley',

Follows behind the inner ankle, to separate out and enter into the
    heel.

Thereby it ascends inside the calf to come out at the inner edge of
    the back of the knee,

Travelling upwards along the inner back edge of the thigh,

Passing directly through the backbone,

To belong to the Kidneys and connect up with the Bladder.

It travels directly up from the Kidneys, passing through the Liver
    and diaphragm, to enter into the Lungs,

Following the throat to nestle under the tongue.

A branch comes out from the Lungs to connect up with the Heart

And pour into the 'middle chest'.

心主手厥陰心包絡之脈, 起於胸中, 出屬心胞絡, 下膈歷絡三焦.
其支者, 循胸出脅, 下腋三寸, 上抵腋, 下循臑內行太陰少陰之間入肘中,
下臂行兩筋之間入掌中, 循中指出其端.
其支者, 別掌中循小指次指出其端.

THE HEART LORD HAND JUEYIN is the 'connector' vessel,

Which embraces the heart, rising up from the 'middle chest'.

It comes out, belonging to the 'connector' which embraces the
    heart,

Travelling down to the diaphragm, successively passing through
    the *Sanjiao*.

A branch follows the chest, coming out at the ribs,

At a point three inches under the armpit,

Travelling upwards to reach under the armpit,

Following the inside of the upper arm,

Passing between the Taiyin and Shaoyin, to enter into the elbow,
Travelling down the forearm, to pass between the two tendons,
And enter into the midst of the palm, where it follows the middle
    finger to come out at its tip.

Another branch separates out from the midst of the palm,
To follow the finger next to the little finger to come out at its tip.

三焦手少陽之脈, 起於小指次指之端, 上出兩指之間.
循手表腕出臂外兩骨之間, 上貫肘, 循臑外上肩而交出足少陽之後,
入缺盆, 布膻中, 散絡心胞, 下膈循屬三焦.
其支者, 從膻中上出缺盆, 上項系耳後直上出耳上角, 以屈下頰出頤.
其支者, 從耳後入耳中, 出走耳前, 過客主人前, 交頰至目銳眦.

THE *SANJIAO* HAND SHAOYANG VESSEL rises from the tip
    of the finger next to the little finger and travels up,
Coming out in the space between the two fingers.
It follows the hand along the outer wrist,
Coming out on the outer forearm between the two bones,
And travels up, passing directly through the elbow,
Follows the outer side of the upper arm, to travel up to the
    shoulder,
Crossing and coming out behind the foot Shaoyang,
Enters into the 'broken basin', spreading into the middle of the
    chest,
To scatter and connect up with the vessel which embraces the
    heart,
Travelling down to the diaphragm, and following on to belong to
    the *Sanjiao*.

Another branch, from the middle of the chest, travels up to come
    out at the 'broken basin',
Travels up beside the nape of the neck, behind the ear,
Travelling straight upwards to come out at the upper corner of
    the ear,
Thence bending down to the cheekbone to arrive at under the eyes.

Another branch, from behind the ear,
Enters into the ear and comes out,

Running in front of the ear, passing across the 'guest and host' in
    front,
To cross over the cheek and arrive at the outer corner of the eye.

膽足少陽之脈, 起於目銳眥, 上抵頭角, 下耳後, 循頸.
行手少陽之前至肩上, 卻交出手少陽之後入缺盆.
其支者, 從耳後入耳中, 出走耳前至目銳眥後.
其支者, 別銳眥下大迎, 合於手少陽, 抵於䪼, 下加頰車, 下頸合缺盆,
以下胸中, 貫膈絡肝屬膽, 從脅裡出氣街, 繞毛際橫入髀厭中.
以下循髀陽出膝外廉, 下外輔骨之前, 直下抵絕骨之端,
下出外踝之前, 循足跗上入小指次指之間.
其支者, 別跗上入大指間, 循大指岐骨內出其端, 還貫爪甲出三毛.

THE GALLBLADDER FOOT SHAOYANG VESSEL rises at
    the outer corner of the eye,
Travels up to reach the corner of the head and then down behind
    the ear and follows the neck,
Passing in front of the hand Shaoyang, to arrive at the shoulder,
Turns back and crosses over to come out behind the hand
    Shaoyang and enter the 'broken basin'.
A branch, from behind the ear, enters into the ear,
Comes out, running in front of the ear, to arrive behind the
    corner of the eye.

Another branch separates out at the corner of the eye,
Travels down to 'great welcome',
Then reunites with the hand Shaoyang, to reach under the eyes,
Travelling down once more to the 'jawbone joint', to reunite at
    the 'broken basin'.
Thereby it travels down the 'middle chest',
Passing directly through the diaphragm,
To connect up with the Liver and belong to the Gallbladder,
Following the lining of the ribs to come out at the 'qi highway',
Entwining the region of hair and horizontally entering into the
    hip joint.
It travels directly from the 'broken basin' under by the armpit,
Following within the chest, passing across the floating ribs, down
    to reunite at the hip joint,
Thereby it follows down the Yang portion of the thigh,

Coming out at the outer edge of the knee,

Travelling down in front of the outer 'supporting bone',

Passing directly down to reach the tip of the 'terminate bone',

Travelling down to come out before the outer ankle,

Following the top of the instep, to enter into the tip of the toe
     next to the little toe.

Another branch separates out at the instep, to enter into the gap
     by the big toe,

And follows along inside the bone of the big toe to come out at
     its tip,

Circling back to pass directly through into the nail, and come out
     at its few hairs.

肝足厥陰之脈, 起於大指叢毛之際.

上循足跗上廉, 去內踝一寸, 上踝八寸, 交出太陰之後, 上膕內廉,

循股陰入毛中, 過陰器, 抵小腹, 挾胃屬肝絡膽.

上貫膈, 布脇肋, 循喉嚨之後上入頏顙連目系, 上出額, 與督脈會於巔.

　　其支者, 從目系下頰裡, 環脣內.

其支者, 復從肝別貫膈, 上注肺.

THE LIVER FOOT JUEYIN VESSEL rises in the region of the
     bunch of hair on the big toe.

It travels upwards following the upper surface of the instep,

One inch away from the inside ankle,

Travels up to eight inches above the ankle, to cross over and come
     out behind the Taiyin,

Travelling up the inside edge of the hollow behind the knee,

Following the inner thigh, to enter into the middle of the hair,

Passing over the sex organs, to reach the lower belly,

Travelling alongside the stomach, to belong to the Liver and
     connect up with the Gallbladder.

It then travels upwards, passing through the diaphragm, to spread
     into the ribs,

Following behind the throat, upwards to enter in where the nose
     joins the back of the throat,

To link up with the system of the eyes,

Travelling up to come out at the forehead, and then meet with the
     Governor vessel at the crown.

A branch, from the system of the eyes,

Travels down the lining of the cheek, to ring around inside the
  lips.

Another branch, again from the Liver, passes separately through
  the diaphragm,

Afterwards travelling upwards to pour into the Lungs.

任脈者, 起於中極之下, 以上毛際,

循腹裡上關元, 至咽喉, 上頤, 循面入目.

THE CONCEPTION VESSEL rises at a point beneath the
  'central pole',

Thereby travelling up and over the hair border,

Following the lining of the belly, to travel up to 'pass primal' to
  arrive at the throat,

Travels up by the lower chin, to follow across the face and enter
  into the eyes.

督脈起於少腹以下骨中央, 女子入系廷孔. 其孔, 溺孔之端也.

其絡循陰器合篡間, 繞篡後, 別繞臀至少陰,

與巨陽中絡者合少陰上股內後廉, 貫脊屬腎.

與太陽起於目內眥, 上額交巔上, 入絡腦, 還出別下項, 循脊抵腰中,

入循脊絡腎. 其男子循莖下至篡, 與女子等.

其少腹直上者, 貫齊中央, 上貫心, 入喉上頤環唇, 上系兩目之下中央.

THE GOVERNOR VESSEL rises at the lower belly

To travel down into the bony central region.

In a woman it enters in and ties up with the front opening, the
  tip of the urine-hole.

It connects up with and follows the sexual organs,

Reuniting at the 'crossing space' and twining around behind the
  'crossing space',

To separately entwine the buttocks, arrives at the Shaoyin,

Connecting up with the Huge Yang, reuniting with the Shaoyin
  above,

By travelling up the inner back edge of the thigh,

To pass directly through the backbone to belong to the Kidneys.

Along with the Taiyang it rises at the inner corner of the eye,
Travelling up and over the forehead, to cross over at the crown,
Travelling up to enter in and connect up with the brain,
Circling back to come out separately down the nape of the neck,
Following the shoulder, inside the shoulder blade,
Besides the backbone reaching down into the waist,
To enter in and follow the spine to connect up with the Kidneys.
In a male it follows down the stem of the penis to arrive at the
    'crossing', the same as in a woman.

From the lower belly it travels up directly,
Passing through the 'central region' at the navel,
Travelling up directly through the heart to enter into the throat,
And passing upward on over the chin to ring the lips,
Reaching up, to tie up with the 'central region' beneath both eyes.

This chapter contains the text describing the channels taken directly from *Lingshu*. It is the oldest source for the twelve Jingluo 經絡, beginning with the Lung hand Taiyin, then progressing through the hand and foot Yangming, foot Taiyin, hand Shaoyin, foot Taiyang, foot Shaoyin, hand Jueyin, hand and foot Shaoyang, and foot Taiyin, ending up with the two extra channels, the Du and Ren. The origin, direction, main pathway and subsequent branches of each channel are meticulously described. The text carries considerable sophistication. Many technical terms are used to convey the subtleties of channel identification. These include: rises (*qi* 起); connects up (*luo* 絡); belong to (*shu* 屬); comes out (*chu* 出); follows (*xun* 循); travelling, passing (*xing* 行); enter in (*ru* 入); straight, directly, travelling on (*zhi* 直); passing through (*guan* 貫); alongside, beside, nestling (*xie* 挾); crossing over, passing across (*jiao* 交); ringing (*huan* 環); passing over (*guo* 過); arrive at (*zhi* 至); reach down/under (*di* 抵); separately (*bie* 別); scatter (*san* 散); pour into (*zhu* 注); entwines (*rao* 繞); slant-wise (*xie* 斜); bending down (*qu* 屈); reunites (*he* 合); and spreads (*bu* 布). I have tried to remain true to the character of the text, using the simple Saxon English to avoid 'westernising' with modern anatomy. Named acupoints and a few landmarks are identified in the notes.

The *Sanjiao* 三焦 is the channel joining the three heating-spaces of the body – thorax, middle diaphragm and lower belly.

Note that, in this early text, both deep and superficial pathways of the linking network are recorded together. There was no initial separation. The surface recognition of points probably followed on – due to their efficacy. Note also that the branching of each channel is indicated. There is always an emphasis on function. Xue Shengbai comments on this description of the pathways:

> The whole set of twenty-seven qi arises like a flowing spring of water, resting neither by night nor day. The Yin vessels nourish the five *zang*, the Yang vessels nourish the six *fu*; in the end they return to the beginning, forming a continuous cycle, without a break. The proper channels are similar to irrigation canals or ditches, whilst the extra channels form the wetlands and tidal marshes. Take as a picture the falling rain, filling the ditches and then flowing on into and irrigating the wetlands and tidal marshes. As the *zangfu* represent the roots of the Jingluo, so the Jingluo become their stalks and leaves. Become well acquainted with the Jingluo, and the *yinyang*, outer and inner, qi and blood, *xu* weak and *shi* strong will be taken into your heart, to nestle there. If you are a beginner, first attend to the facts in front of your face – there is no divine skill that lies beyond them. The rough worker acts blindly, and his false words hit wide of the mark. The wise scholar examines precisely what he sees – he responds only by adapting his work tirelessly to what is in front of him, to the situation at hand.

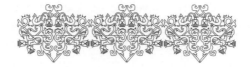

Question for Review of Chapter VI

1. Giving as much detail as you can, list the pathways of any three channels on the body. Be sure to include deep pathways as well.

Characters in Chapter VI

channels 經絡 *Jingluo*

rises 起 *qi*

connects up 絡 *luo*

belongs to 屬 *shu*

comes out 出 *chu*

follows 循 *xun*

travelling, passing 行 *xing*

enters in 入 *ru*

straight, directly, travelling on 直 *zhi*

passing through 貫 *guan*

alongside, beside, nestling 挾 *xie*

crossing over, passing across 交 *jiao*

ringing 環 *huan*

passing over 過 *guo*

arrives at 至 *zhi*

reach down/under 抵 *di*

separately 別 *bie*

scatter 散 *san*

pour into 注 *zhu*

entwines 繞 *rao*

slant-wise 斜 *xie*

bending down 屈 *qu*

reunites 合 *he*

spreads 布 *bu*

three-heater 三焦 *Sanjiao*

VII

Patterns of Treatment

As is well known, when a workman sets out to
build a carriage, he selects a set-square and pair of
compasses. He does not rely on human skill alone.

Key Ideas

1. *Yin and Yang, the Rule and Pattern*
   Yin and Yang, their resonance, 'a clear mind', seeking the
   root

2. *The Seed in Sickness*
   seeking the root, the *shi* strong (full), *xu* empty (weak), the
   wuxing, balance

3. *Mind, Body and Disease*
   the appropriateness of each medicine, moxa and needle,
   stone probes, hot compresses, *daoyin*, herbal brews,
   rubbing, massage

4. *Regional Types, Regional Medicines*
   the peoples of the different regions, appropriate (best)
   treatment, the work of the ancient Sages, different methods,
   stone probes, 'poison herbs', moxa, fine needle, *daoyin*
   (massage), all have one aim

5. *Treatment with Herbals, Foodstuffs and Flavours*
   Yin and Yang, the pungent, sweet, salty, sour and fragrant, their actions, balance, to accord with the condition, returning aback, overuse

6. *How Foodstuffs and Medicines can do Harm*
   the overuse of both foodstuffs and medicines

7. *Therapeutic Actions, How to Treat*
   let them be appropriate, herbal action, strong and weak conditions

8. *Five Faults Made during Treatment*
   not to know the emotional background to the disease, not to read the classics, not to identify 'loss of esteem', the rough physician

9. *The Ultimate Task*
   colour and pulse, negligence, the real substance, find the first cause, the spirit

Some questions for review can be found at the end of this chapter.

1. Yin and Yang, the Rule and Pattern

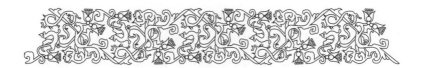

陰陽者天地之道也.

萬物之綱紀也, 變化之父母, 生殺之本始, 神明之府也.

治病必求於本.

THE YIN AND YANG FORM THE WAY of the skies and
    earth;
They make up the rules and pattern for all myriad creatures.
They are the father and mother
Of all change and transformation,
The root origin of living and killing,
The treasury of a clear mind.
To heal sickness you must seek out their root.

Li Zhongzi: This explains how Heaven and Earth, all myriad things, change
and transformation, living and killing, all lie nowhere but in the Yin and Yang.
Examine them precisely and you should be able to meet up with a clear mind.
Thus when first coming upon and treating an illness, there appear ten thousand
loose ends, all tangled up and confused – but from them you must seek out the
root 本 ben. Sickness either originates in the Yin or in the Yang. Once Yin and
Yang have been determined, all sickness and calamity fly away.

The Huainan Zi: The double purity of the skies and earth forms the Yin and
Yang; the single purity of Yin and Yang forms the four seasons; the scattered
purity of the seasons forms all the myriad creatures.

Yin and Yang again head up this chapter – but in the next few
selections they are pursued in detail. These few lines describe

the overwhelming character of the *yinyang*. Li Zhongzi's earlier commentary explains the full implication of 'the root' 本 *ben*:

> All humankind is beset by sickness. Although it has no single cause, sickness either belongs to the category of the weak (*xu*) or strong (*shi*), to cold or heat, to qi or blood, to *zang* or *fu*, and all these are contained within the Yin and Yang. For that reason, although our understanding of sickness alters constantly, Yin and Yang remain the root.

Be clear in diagnosis and treatment: this is a prerequisite for understanding 'the single idea', and results in the best treatment. This relates to Yang Wangming's take on 'the extension of knowledge through the investigation of things' in the Introduction. The lines above on the *yinyang* are rightly famous as they open our eyes to the 'basic and grand simplicity' (太素 *taisu*) of the *Neijing*'s approach.

THE YIN AND YANG

the Way	of the skies and earth
the rules and pattern	for all myriad creatures
the father and mother	all change and transformation
the root origin	of living and killing
the treasury	of a clear mind

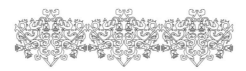

2. The Seed in Sickness

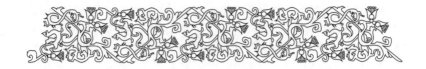

謹守病機, 各司其屬. 有者求之, 無者求之. 盛者責之, 虛者責之.
必先五勝, 疏其血氣, 令其調達, 而致和平.

REVERENTLY DETERMINE THE SEED of the sickness;
Manage each occurrence according to kind.
If there is something apparent, then seek it out.
If there is nothing apparent – then also seek this out.
If it is full, you should deal with it.
If it is weak, you should also deal with it.
You must first make use of the 'five prevailing forces'.
Ease the flow of the qi and blood to make them expansive.
Then the condition will balance out and the patient finds peace.

Zhang Jiebin: If there is 'something apparent', it means a *shi* strong condition; if there is 'nothing apparent', it means a *xu* weak condition. To 'seek it out' means to seek out the root, that which is actually there, it is either something or nothing.

Wang Bing: When the heart is full, it produces heat; when the kidneys are full, they produce cold. If the kidneys are weak, the cold moves within; if the heart is weak, the heat retreats inside. In the same manner a heat which cannot be cooled is a 'no water' situation; and a cold which cannot be warmed is a 'no fire' situation. This is a cold which is 'not a cold' and you deal with it as a 'no fire' situation; and this is a heat which is 'not a heat' and you deal with it as a 'no water' situation. A heat which does not last, you deal with as a weakness of the heart; a cold which does not last, you deal with as a shortage in the kidneys. If there is something apparent, you drain it; if there is nothing apparent, you reinforce. If there is weakness, you reinforce. If there is fullness, you drain.

The Yin and Yang, in treatment and practice, govern everything. They particularly encompass all intricacies of medical thinking which eventually result in a 'clear mind' 神明 *shenming*. All aspects of sickness, diagnosis, needling and prescribing yield to their practicality, often with astonishing results. We are admonished to 'reverently determine the seed of the sickness', as illness can occur in countless forms, all of which should be examined carefully in order to gain a clear understanding of contradiction in symptomology. This is why I have appended Wang Bing's thorny comment above. But none of this lies beyond an analysis in terms of Yin and Yang, the apparent, or not apparent – a 'full, strong, real' 實 *shi* or 'weak, empty, deficient' 虛 *xu* condition. The 'five prevailing forces' – cycles of wood, earth, fire, water and metal qi and their procession – determine the balance in health and disease. The 'seed' or 'causative factor' 機 *ji* stirs as a motivating force – from which we may command any action. But if we are to be both accommodating and alive in examination and treatment, we must make use of the whole of the *yinyang*. A full condition may appear as empty, and an empty condition may appear as full. In conditions of weakness, *xu* can masquerade as *shi*, and *shi* as *xu*. There can occur a 'cold' which is 'not a cold' and a 'heat' which is 'not a heat'. So then we use gentle tonics on either the kidneys or heart, accordingly. The most common example of this would be the hot 'night-sweats' during a woman's menopause, or after a severe illness. This is 'empty fire' on the outside – due to long-term weakness within – and, in some cases, it should not be dealt with by the use of cooling medicines but paradoxically by gentle, heating tonics. This is what is meant by 'to manage each occurrence according to kind'. This matter is also covered by Section 5 when using 'cold medicines to treat a hot sickness, and hot medicines to treat a cold sickness'.

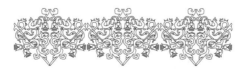

3. Mind, Body and Disease

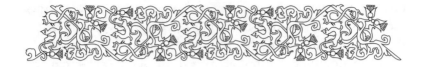

形樂志苦, 病生於脈, 治之以灸刺.
形樂志樂, 病生於肉, 治之以鍼石.
形苦志樂, 病生於筋, 治之以熨引.
形苦志苦, 病生於咽嗌, 治之以百藥.
形數驚恐, 經絡不通, 病生於不仁, 治之以按摩醪藥.

THE BODY WELL but the mind suffering,
The disease is born in the vessels;
You heal it using moxa and needle.
The body well and the mind well,
The disease is born in the flesh;
You heal it using stone probes.
The body suffering but the mind well,
The disease is born in the tendons;
You heal it using hot compresses and *daoyin*.
The body suffering and the mind suffering,
Disease is born in the throat and insides,
You heal it using all kinds of herbals.
The body in a great deal of terror and fright,
The Jingluo not moving well at all.
This disease is born from a lack of sensation in the muscles.
You heal it using rubbing, massage and herbal brews.

This section shows the appropriateness of each medicine to each condition. The compresses would have been made with herbal brews, clay and mud, and possibly also hot stones or 'ironing' applied to the body. *Daoyin* implies rubbing and massage, or even calisthenics. Note how the location of the disease is identified in each case and subsequently an appropriate therapy applied. Causes are astutely recognised and removed. I have followed the SWYS text in this section, as the NJZY does not include it.

PROPRIETY OF THE CURE

body and mind	disease	to heal
body well, mind suffering	born in the vessels	using moxa and needle
body well, mind well	born in the flesh	using stone probes
body suffering, mind well	born in the tendons	using hot compresses and daoyin
body suffering, mind suffering	in the throat and insides	using all kinds of herbals

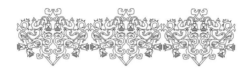

4. Regional Types, Regional Medicines

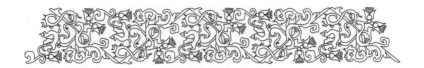

故東方之域, 天地之所始生也, 魚鹽之地, 海濱傍水.

其民食魚而嗜鹹, 皆安其處.

美其食, 魚者使人熱中, 鹽者勝血.

故其民皆黑色疎理, 其病皆為癰瘍.

其治宜砭石, 故砭石者, 亦從東方來.

IN THE OUTER LANDS TO THE EAST, heaven and earth
first come into being.

It is a land of fish, and briny waters,

Being close to the regions of the sea.

Its people eat fish and salty things, but are always peaceful in their
homes.

They enjoy their food, but the fish causes them to retain heat
within.

The saltiness attacks the blood.

So these people all show a darkened skin.

As it breaks up within, their diseases are all ulcers and boils.

They can best be treated by stone probes.

Therefore stone probes are commonly used in the outer lands to
the east.

西方者, 金玉之域, 沙石之處.

天地之所收引也. 其民陵居而多風, 水土剛強.

其民不衣而褐薦, 其民華食而脂肥, 故邪不能傷其形體, 其病生於內.

其治宜毒藥. 故毒藥者, 亦從西方來.

To the west are the outer lands of gold and gems.

This is a place of coarse sands and stones.

It is where heaven and earth close and draw in.

Its people dwell in the hills and it is often windy, the waters and
soils are hard and difficult to till.

They do not dress fine but wear wool, and sleep on mats.

But they eat well and become fat and overweight.

Therefore the malign *xie* does not injure their outer form – and
disease is born within.

They can be best treated with 'poison herbs'.

Therefore 'poison herbs' are commonly used in western lands.

北方者, 天地所閉藏之域也, 其地高陵居, 風寒冰冽.

其民樂野處而乳食, 藏寒生滿病.

其治宜灸焫. 故灸焫者, 亦從北方來.

To the north, heaven and earth reveal a landscape that is closed up
and hidden.

It is a land of high peaks, the wind blows cold,

With ice and freezing conditions.

So its people make merry in the wilderness by eating milk
products.

The stored-up cold produces a full type of disease.

They are best healed with the burning of moxa.

Therefore burning moxa is commonly used in northern lands.

南方者, 天地所長養, 陽之所盛處也.

其地下, 水土弱, 霧露之所聚也.

其民嗜酸而食胕故其民皆緻理而赤色, 其病攣痹.

其治宜微鍼. 故九鍼者, 亦從南方來.

In southern areas, heaven and earth broaden out and the land is
productive,

It is warm with expansive areas.

The land is lower, the waters and soils softer,

And fogs and mists tend to gather.

So its people consume pickles and dried meats.

They are all more delicate within, with reddened skins.

They complain of spasms, numbness and *bi* immobility.

They are best treated with the very fine needle.

Therefore this kind of needle is commonly used in southern lands.

中央者, 其地平以濕, 天地所以生萬物也眾.

其民食雜而不勞, 故其病多痿厥寒熱.

其治宜導引按蹻. 故導引按蹻者, 亦從中央出也.

In the central regions, here the land is flatter and damper.

This is where heaven and earth produce a multitude of creatures.

The people there eat all kinds of foodstuffs, and the living is easy.

Therefore when they fall sick it is often with wasting and reverse-
flowing fevers.

They are best treated with *daoyin* rubbing, pressing and massage.

Therefore rubbing, pressing and massage are more common in
central regions.

故聖人雜合以治, 各得其所宜, 故治所以異而病皆愈者.

得病之情, 知治之大體也.

Therefore the Sages had but one single aim, but used various
methods to heal.

Each time they accorded with what was fitting.

In treatment there are differing methods – but the aim is always
to cure.

To obtain the background condition of the disease

Is to understand the main body of our work in treatment.

The last two lines of this passage summarise its message. To obtain the 'background condition' 情 *qing* ('emotion, feeling, situation') of the disease will yield the appropriate treatment. In Section 8 below, 'Five Faults Made during Treatment', this concept is extended to include emotional factors.

When the patient walks into the consulting room, an understanding of the greater picture allows us to tailor the treatment to the individual. Each person thrives in a distinct and differing environment, differing even from that of a close neighbour. In each of the five directions (east, west, south, north, central) a separate landscape appears: followed by people with differing habits and diets. Note the importance of diet. Each presenting patient should be accorded the best possible treatment – that which is suited to the illness and its cause. This section illustrates how variability may arise in medical practice, although the Sages 'had but one single aim, to cure'; that is, to tailor the medicine to the region and to the type of person inhabiting that region. Thus medicine becomes truly person-centred. Traditional Chinese medicine was primarily local, folk medicine.

TREATMENTS TAILORED TO LOCALITY AND BACKGROUND

direction	the land	the people	their illnesses	best treated
to the east	is of fish and briny waters, close to regions of the sea	eat fish and salty things, but are peaceful in their homes	heat retained within, the saltiness attacks the blood, ulcers and boils	by stone probes
to the west	of gold and gems, coarse sands and stones	dress fine, wear wool, sleep on mats, eat well	become fat and overweight, the malign *xie* born within, not without	with 'poison herbs'
to the north	is closed up and hidden, of high peaks, the wind cold	make merry in the wilderness, by eating milk products	stored-up cold produces a full type of disease	with burning moxa
in southern areas	is broader and productive, warm, with fogs and mists	consume pickles, dried meats, are delicate within, with red skins	complain of spasms, numbness and *bi* immobility	with a very fine needle
in central regions	is flatter and damper, and the living is easy	eat all kinds of foodstuffs, and the living is easy	fall sick, often with wasting and reverse-flowing fevers	with *daoyin* rubbing, pressing and massage

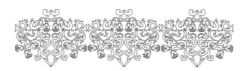

5. Treatment with Herbals, Foodstuffs and Flavours

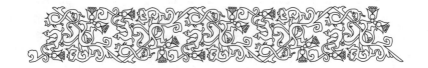

帝曰: 善. 五味陰陽之用何如? 岐伯曰:
辛甘發散為陽, 酸苦涌泄為陰, 鹹味涌泄為陰, 淡味滲泄為陽.
六者或收或散, 或緩或急, 或燥或潤或軟或堅.

THE YELLOW EMPEROR SAID: Good, now how are the five
flavours applied in terms of Yin and Yang? And Qi Bo answers:
Pungent and sweet flavours express and disperse and are Yang.
Sour and bitter flavours may gush out and dissipate and are Yin.
Salty flavours may gush out and dissipate and are Yin.
Bland flavours permeate and dissipate and are Yang.
These six are either astringent or dispersing,
Either slowing down or hastening,
Either drying out or moistening,
Either softening or hardening.

以所利而行之, 調其氣使其平也.
Use those most favourable and those which work,
To harmonise the qi and bring it into balance.

Li Zhongzi: To 'gush out' means to work as an emetic. To 'dissipate' means
to purge.

寒者熱之, 熱者寒之, 微者逆之, 甚者從之, 堅者削之, 客者除之,
勞者溫之, 結者散之, 留者攻之, 燥者濡之, 急者緩之, 散者收之.
損者溫之, 逸者行之, 驚者平之,

上之下之, 摩之浴之, 薄之劫之,
開之發之, 適事為故.

If they are cold, then heat them.

If they are hot, then cool them down.

If the condition is slight, you can work against it.

If it is severe, then go along with it.

Where there is hardness, split it apart.

If the qi inhabits within, throw it out.

If it is overworked, gently warm it.

When the qi is getting in a knot, disperse it.

As it is lingering, attack it.

As it is dried up, dampen it.

If it quickens, slow it down.

If it is dispersing, use astringents.

If lessening, add to it.

If idling, put it to work.

If startled, pacify it.

When it rises above, bring it down.

Massage it, bathe it, thin it out,

Break it apart, open it out and help it express itself.

All actions must accord with the condition.

Li Zhongzi: 'All actions must accord with the condition. ' In other words, measure what degree of sickness is present, and act to halt it. Neither go on too long with the treatment so as to injure their health, nor undertreat and end up retaining the malign *xie*.

逆者正治, 從者反治. 從少從多, 觀其事也.

To go against it, means to properly treat it.

To go along with it, means to contrarily treat it.

Whether you go along with it, employing the lesser ingredient,

Or go along with it, employing the greater ingredient,

Observe each occurrence according to its state.

Li Zhongzi: To 'go along with it, employing the lesser ingredient' means one part of the medicine goes along with the condition and two parts go against it. To 'go along with it, employing the greater ingredient' means two parts of the medicine go along with the condition and one part goes against. The 'state' is the particular state of the illness. Observe the severity of each occurrence of the sickness, personally making up a prescription with greater or lesser quantities.

熱因寒用, 寒因熱用.

Heat is employed in cold conditions,
Cold is employed in hot conditions.

Li Zhongzi: In a cold sickness, employ heat, but when the cold is severe, limit the heat. You must use hot medicines, taken down cold. In a hot sickness, employ cold, but when the heat is severe, limit the cold. You must use cold medicines, taken down hot.

塞因塞用, 通因通用.

In stagnancy, employ the stagnancy,
When flowing freely, employ the free-flowing.

Li Zhongzi: In stagnancy, 'employ the stagnancy' refers, for instance, to when the middle *jiao* is blocked due to weak and failing qi. You want to disperse the fullness but you will further weaken the failing qi; you want to reinforce the failing qi but the fullness within will increase. So then, treat without taking notice of the root condition, by first attacking the fullness. The medicine taken down will perhaps diminish it. But if the medicine is carried on too long, the patient will further weaken. Then the sickness will transmit on and worsen. If you do not know to reduce the dose, the condition will block up further. Increase the dose, until it reaches through and flows freely. Working in such a skilled manner, you reinforce the failing qi and the weak get stronger of their own accord while the fullness moves on, also of its own accord.

必伏其所主, 而先其所因, 其始則同, 其終則異,
可使破積, 可使潰堅, 可使氣和, 可使必已.

You must overcome the main part! But prioritise the cause.
At the beginning they look the same, in the end they diverge.
You can break up any accumulation,
You can break apart the hard,
You can pacify the energies.
If you can do it, you must finish it!

Ma Shi: Whatever is the 'main part' (主 *zhu*) of the body of the disease, you must have the appetite to overcome it. For instance, 'using heat to treat cold conditions, and cold to treat hot conditions'. Use whichever herb is suitable.

This is the one you must put first. For instance, 'knowing that the cause lies in cold, or heat, or stagnancy or the "free-flowing"'.

Li Zhongzi: 'To overcome the main part' means to be sharp as to the root of the illness; 'to prioritise the cause' means to seek out its cause. 'At the beginning they look the same' describes 'properly' treating the condition, or 'contrarily' going against it. 'In the end they diverge' describes 'contrarily' treating the condition, or 'properly' going along with it. If you understand this method of 'contrarily' treating a condition, there is no sickness which will not heal!

諸寒之而熱者取之陰, 熱之而寒者取之陽, 所謂求其屬也.

In all cold conditions which produce heat, select the Yin.

In all hot conditions which produce cold, select the Yang.

This is what is meant by 'seek out according to kind'.

Li Zhongzi: When you use cold medicines to treat a hot sickness, but instead the heat increases, this is not a fire which is excessive but a Yin which is insufficient. If Yin is insufficient the fire may become over-strong, so medicines for the Yin should be used. Only tonify the Yin, and the Yang withdraws naturally. And when you use hot medicines to treat a cold sickness, but instead the cold increases, this is not a cold which is excessive but a Yang which is insufficient. If Yang is insufficient there may be Yin cold, so medicines for the Yang should be employed. Only reinforce the 'fire in the water', and the cold naturally disperses. 'To seek out according to kind' means seeking out the root of the sickness. A single water and a single fire, both may be sought in the kidneys. Thus Wang, our Great Teacher, said: 'Increase the source of the fire, thus to disperse the Yin gloom! Strengthen the ruling water, thus to control the bright Yang!' The six-flavoured pill (*Liuwei Dihuang*) and the eight-flavoured pill (*Bawei Dihuang*), these two medicines are all you need.

All signs and symptoms, diagnoses and patterns of treatment are interrelated. Tastes and flavours, foods and medicine, all have a particular character or nature 性 *xing* – either Yin or Yang. Pungent and sweet flavours disperse, sour and bitter gush out, and so on. All the other flavours work accordingly. Furthermore, each herb and foodstuff has its own particular action. They can slow down or hasten, dry out or moisten, soften or harden, and so on. There is a concrete logic to this approach. In treatment we plainly use that which is appropriate, that 'which accords with the condition'. Yet there is a warning here. As Li Zhongzi stresses, neither 'go on too long, so as to injure the healthy state' (this is especially the case with herbal medication), nor 'undertreat and end up retaining the malign *xie*'.

Regulation and harmony are to the fore. Use medicines most suited to the time and place. You may perhaps take heating medicines cold, or else cooling medicines warmed. This will ameliorate their action. In cases of stagnancy, go first for the root condition. But do not continue this treatment too long. As the condition changes, you should alter the prescription. This is the meaning of 'when stagnant, employ the stagnancy; when flowing freely, employ the free-flowing'. You treat each situation, each moment, again 'according to kind'.

To 'overcome the main part' 伏其所主 *fu qisuo zhu* and to 'prioritise the cause' 先其所因 *xian qisuo yin* refers to attacking the sickness at root. You may act 'properly' 正 *zheng*; you may act 'contrarily' 反 *fan*. In other words: 'Do you heat, do you cool?' It all depends on the immediate situation – and this changes.

We work to moderate their qi and level it out. If they are cool, then heat them; if they are hot, then cool them. This is certainly 'not rocket science'. However, beware contradictory conditions: hot conditions may appear cool, and cold conditions as heated. In both cases you perhaps 'go along with' 從 *cong* or 'go against' 逆 *ni* what you see – sometimes even doing both at once; that is, putting both warming and cooling ingredients in the same mix. Every situation is different, so we need careful scrutiny and observation coupled with direct thought: treating each 'according to kind'. Their rules and patterns demand careful study, especially for herbal practitioners. The distinctions and divisions made above are quite subtle.

HERBAL ACTIONS MUST ACCORD

flavour	action	Yin and Yang
pungent and sweet	express and disperse	Yang
sour and bitter	gush out and dissipate	Yin
salty	gush out and dissipate	Yang
bland	permeate and dissipate	Yin

ACTING IN ACCORD WITH THE CONDITION

condition	action
cold	heat them
hot	cool them down
slight	work against it
severe	go along with it
inhabiting within	throw it out
overworked	gently warm
in a knot	disperse them
lingering	attack them
dried up	dampen them
quickening	slow them down
dispersing	use astringents
lessening	add to them
idling	put them to work
startled	pacify them
rise above	bring them down
cold conditions	use heat
hot conditions	use cold
stagnancy	employ the stagnancy
flowing freely	employ the free-flowing

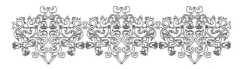

6. How Foodstuffs and Medicines can do Harm

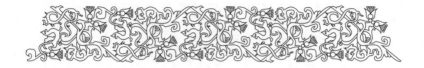

夫五味入胃, 各歸所喜攻.

AS TO THE FIVE FLAVOURS entering the stomach,
Each 'returns aback' to its organ
Where it either does harm or good.

酸先入肝, 苦先入心, 甘先入脾, 辛先入肺, 鹹先入腎.
久而增氣, 物化之常也. 氣增而久, 夭之由也.

Sourness initially enters the liver,
Bitterness initially enters the heart,
Sweetness initially enters the spleen,
Pungency initially enters the lungs,
Saltiness initially enters the kidneys.
Taken over a long period of time they will benefit the qi:
This is the usual way in which things grow and transform.
But once these tastes have benefited the organs and they continue
     to be taken,
They become a sure cause of early death.

All foodstuffs, flavours and medicines can benefit the *zangfu*
organs; but taken over a long period of time, such as in long-term
prescribing or a mono-diet, they can also harm and cause damage.
They can even be a cause of premature death.

7. Therapeutic Actions, How to Treat

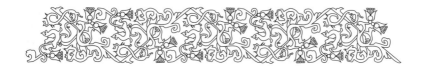

因其輕而揚之, 因其重而減之, 因其衰而彰之.

形不足者, 溫之以氣, 精不足, 補之以味.

TAKE THAT WHICH IS LIGHT, and bring it out accordingly.

Take that which is severe, and reduce it, accordingly.

Take that which is weakened and manifest it, accordingly.

When the body is not strong, build it up through its qi.

When the *jing* is not strong, tonify it with flavours.

其高者, 因而越之, 其下者, 引而竭之, 中滿者瀉之於內.

其有邪者, 漬形以為汗, 其在皮者, 汗而發之.

其慄悍者, 按而收之, 其實者散而瀉之.

When they are high up, go along with them and let them
   encroach.

When they are below, guide them down and exhaust them.

When they are blocked inside, clear them out from within.

Where there is malign *xie*, soak it out as sweat.

When it lies in the skin, create a sweat and express it.

If the condition is sudden or fierce, halt it using astringents.

If it is strong, then disperse and drain it.

Li Zhongzi: High up means you are sick in the upper *jiao*. To 'encroach' means
to vomit up. They encroach and rise up. Below means you are sick in the lower
jiao. To 'exhaust' means to send out below. Guide the qi and fluids out below.
You help by promoting the working of the two conveniences; both should

be right. Some are of the opinion that to 'guide' means to use sweet honey or bitter medicine as a guide. To 'soak' means to saturate. For instance, select peach twigs to encourage a sweat, or else use a warm broth as an infusion, or else clear the malign *xie* 邪 externally with a double dose. Herbal medicines cannot be used to create a sweat during winter months or cold weather, when to express it is to no avail.

Li Zhongzi: 'Sudden' and hasty, 'fierce' or violent – these are signs of angry qi injuring the liver. To 'halt it' means to control it with sour astringents, for instance medicines such as peony root. If Yin is strong, use cloves, ginger, cinnamon or aconite to scatter the cold; if Yang is strong, scutellaria, coptis root, gardenia fruits or arbor vitae seeds may drain the fire.

審其陰陽, 以別柔剛.

陽病治陰, 陰病治陽. 定其血氣, 各守其鄉.

血實宜決之, 氣虛宜掣引之.

Inspect the Yin and Yang to distinguish the use of firming and
    softening medicines.

When the Yang is sick, treat the Yin.

When the Yin is sick, treat the Yang.

Settle the blood and qi,

Keeping each to its own region.

If the blood is strong, you must undam it.

If the qi is weak, you must pull and lead it along.

Li Zhongzi: If the Yang predominates, it means an injury to the Yin. So treat Yin by reinforcing the ruling water. If Yin predominates, it means an injury to the Yang. So treat Yang by reinforcing the fire within the water (the Yang within the kidneys).

Li Zhongzi: You lift and raise them up, like using your hand to pull something along.

Wang Bing: To 'pull' implies to lead along. To conduct and lead (*daoyin*) so as to track the qi, till it becomes smooth and unimpeded.

This passage concerns mainly herbal therapeutics. The significance of treating appropriately continues. In full and substantive conditions, you must clear out and reduce 瀉 *xie*, while in weak conditions you must reinforce 補 *bu*. Various synonyms are used for these actions. Tastes and flavours can rebuild the constitution ('tonify them with flavours'). Follow each condition, 'according to kind': guide out, clear out, soak, express, astringe, disperse, drain, and so on. This is in very real terms physiotherapy. 'Overcome the main part' *fu qisuo zhu* of the qi, lead it, undam it, settle it, keeping each to its own region. Use both Yin and Yang: do not be rigid. Sometimes clearing, sometimes waiting and tonifying. Wang Bing explains the last line, 'If the qi is weak, you must pull and lead it along', as a clear reference to the Taoist practices of *daoyin* 導引 ('conduct and lead'), the breathing, stretching and rubbing exercises, such as *tai-chi*, which excel in strengthening and rehabilitation. Regulation, moderation and harmony are to the fore.

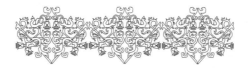

8. Five Faults Made during Treatment

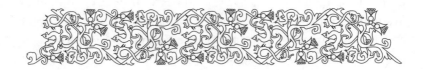

凡未診病者, 必問嘗貴後賤. 雖不中邪, 病從內生, 名曰脫營.

嘗富後貧, 名曰失精, 五氣留連, 病有所并.

良工所失, 不知病情, 此亦治之一過也.

BEFORE YOU COMPLETE THE DIAGNOSIS, ask whether
They were formerly in a honoured position and later demoted.
Even if they have not been hit by any malign *xie* evil,
A disease may have been born inside, due to 'shedding prosperity'.
If they were formerly rich and then poor, this is called 'losing
    worth'.
The five qi connect and linger on, combining to form an illness.
The physician can lose something valuable here.
Not to know the emotional background to the disease is the first
    fault made during treatment.

凡欲診病者, 必問飲食居處, 暴樂暴苦, 始樂後苦, 皆傷精氣.

精氣竭絕, 形體毀沮. 暴怒傷陰, 暴喜傷陽, 厥氣上行, 滿脈去形.

愚醫治之, 不知補寫, 不知病情, 精華日脫, 邪氣乃并,

此治之二過也.

As you are about to make the diagnosis,
You must question as to their diet, and lifestyle.
Do they get sudden peaks of emotion, or are first happy and then
    sink down into despair?
All these can injure the body's essential qi.

As the essential qi is wasted, the body's health declines.

Sudden anger injures the Yin, sudden happiness injures the Yang.

As a rebellious emotion rises, the pulses become full and seem to leave the body.

The physician ignorant of this does not know whether to reinforce or reduce.

He does not understand the emotional background to the illness.

The patient's good health slips away, day by day, and the malign *xie* can take a hold.

This is the second fault made during treatment.

善為脈者, 必以比類奇恒從容知之,
為工而不知道, 此診之不足貴, 此治之三過也.

To be good at holding the pulses, you should be well acquainted with the classical books –

The 'Typography', the 'Strange and Constants' and the 'Habituals'.

A physician who does not know their methods commits the third fault made during treatment.

診有三常, 必問貴賤, 封君敗傷, 及欲侯王.
故貴脫勢, 雖不中邪, 精緻神內傷, 身必敗亡.
始富後貧, 雖不傷邪, 皮焦筋屈, 痿躄為攣.
醫不能嚴, 不能動神, 外為柔弱, 亂至失常.
病不能移, 則醫事不行, 此治之四過也.

During an examination there are three things to observe:

First, determine their position in society,

Second, whether they have commanded respect or met recently with any setback,

And last, whether they have ambition to high rank.

This is because when you lose a valued position,

Although not hit by any malign *xie*, your feelings may be hurt and the self defeated.

Formerly you were rich, now you are poor –

So even though not injured by any malign *xie*, the body may be bent down, and the skin and hair withered.

You may begin to weaken and suffer cramps.

If a physician is not strict about observing these things, he or she
will not enlighten the patient.

They will become less strong, disorder arrives and they lose
constancy.

The disease will not budge and the medicine will be ineffective.

This is the fourth fault made during treatment.

凡風診者, 必知終始, 有知餘緒! 切脈問名, 當合男女.
離絕菀結, 憂恐喜怒, 五藏空虛, 血氣離守. 工不能知, 何術之語?
粗工治之, 亟刺陰陽, 身體解散, 四支轉筋, 死日有期,
醫不能明, 不問所發, 唯言死日, 亦為粗工, 此治之五過也.

When looking at the pathology during an examination, you must
understand it from beginning to end.

In addition you must know that you do not understand
everything!

You must hold the pulse, ask their name, and act appropriately –
whether male or female.

Avoid any confusion or strong emotion in the heart.

You should feel humble and empty, your body calm.

If a physician does not observe in this way, what kind of art is he
practising?

The rough physician pokes at Yin and Yang – and the body is lost
and scattered.

The limbs and tendons unravel, and so he pronounces death is
near – this kind of medicine does nothing.

There is no history. He just blurts out that death is near.

Again this is rough workmanship.

This is the fifth fault made during treatment.

What should be noted here is the importance of understanding
the 'emotional background to the disease' 病情 *bingqing*, of taking
a full history, of pursuing further study of one's art, and the ability
to retain inner composure through the whole of one's work. Then
we may stand a greater chance of avoiding faults.

9. The Ultimate Task

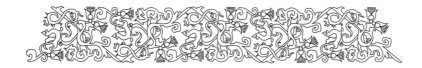

治之要極, 無失色脈,
用之不惑, 治之大則.

THE ULTIMATE TASK IN TREATMENT is not to neglect
colour and pulse.
Make use of them, not to lose them!
This is the great rule in treatment.

逆從到行, 標本不得, 亡神失國. 去故就新, 乃得真.

When forward and backward are confused,
When root and branch cannot be found, you diminish the spirit –
Just as you would neglect a country or state.
'Cast out the old, take in anew. '
Then you can get to the real substance.

歧伯曰: 治之極於一. 一者, 因得之. 帝曰: 奈何?

Qi Bo said: Treatment ultimately comes down to one thing.
That is 'to find out the first cause', then you get the result you
wanted.
The Yellow Emperor said: And how to do it?

歧伯曰: 閉戶塞牖, 繫之病者, 數問其情, 以從其意, 得神者昌, 失神
者亡.

Qi Bo answered:
Close the door and shutter the windows,
Pursue your own ideas on the illness.
Ask all you can about the condition,

Then follow up the main ideas.
If there is spirit, then well and good,
If the spirit has been squandered, the patient is lost.

Zhang Jiebin: That 'one thing' is the root, the first cause that made it all happen. When you find that first cause, then there is nothing you cannot do!

Compare the note to this same passage in Chapter IV, Section 8, 'The Ultimate Tool'. Xue Shengbai comments on this chapter:

The chapters on patterns of treatment have been conveyed to us from the *Neijing* register. While our practice will derive from adapting to circumstances, subtlety comes from our own heart and understanding. Let me explain: do you need to hold up a picture of a horse in front of you, in order to discover a thoroughbred? The pattern will turn and twist in your hand, and you will get lost. There is nothing that cannot be learnt from circumstances! As is well known, when a carpenter sets out to build a carriage, just as others do, he selects a set-square and pair of compasses. He does not rely simply on human skill. Now you can pick up 'the measure of Yin and Yang' and the 'strange and constant' actions of 'the five within'; make decisions from viewing at 'the bright-lit hall' and examine 'the channels' from beginning to end. Then you also may gain the skill of a set-square and pair of compasses!

Questions for Review of Chapter VII
Indicates a more challenging question

1. How does the principle of Yin and Yang apply to 'seeking the root'? Use as a basis for your explanation the separation of 'weak' and 'strong', cold and heat, *zang* and *fu*, and so on.

2. What does Wang Bing mean by a 'no water' and 'no fire' situation? How does fullness masquerade as emptiness?*

3. Give examples of how heat which is 'not a heat' can appear in the body. How would you treat it?

4. What is meant by 'appropriateness' in medicine? Be expansive in your discussion.

5. Describe briefly the five characters of people as illustrated in *Suwen* 12. Then list the five ancient forms of treatment used on each. Why does treatment differ according to people and place?

6. How would you describe the ultimate principle in treating with herbals or diet? Give clinical examples.

7. Describe in detail the actions of 'cold conditions, which produce heat' and 'hot conditions, which produce cold'. How, in brief, would you treat each?*

8. What are the main failings behind the so-called 'five faults' made when treating patients?

Characters in Chapter VII
the root 本 *ben*
basic, the grand simplicity 太素 *taisu*
the clear mind 神明 *shenming*
the apparent condition, full, strong, real 實 *shi*
the apparent condition, weak, empty, deficient 虛 *xu*
causative factor 機 *ji*

background condition, emotion, feeling, situation 情 *qing*

main part 主 *zhu*

a particular character or nature 性 *xing*

overcome the main part 伏其所主 *fu qisuo zhu*

to prioritise the cause (the sickness at root) 先其所因 *xian qisuo yin*

you may act properly 正 *zheng*

you may act contrarily 反 *fan*

go along with the condition 從 *cong*

go against the condition 逆 *ni*

the malign 邪 *xie*

to clear out or reduce in full and substantive conditions 瀉 *xie*

to reinforce in weak conditions 補 *bu*

Taoist practices, breathing, stretching, rubbing exercises 导引 *daoyin*

emotional background to the disease 病情 *bingqing*

VIII

The Method of Needling

When needling...your heart as if approaching
a deep abyss, as if grappling with a tiger!

Key Ideas

1. *Origins of Five Element Acupuncture*
   Yin and Yang, mutual control, the 'five rules', 'simply come,
   simply go', weakness, fullness, the 'minutest of changes'

2. *Opening Chapter of the Lingshu*
   the Yellow Emperor's aim, Qi Bo's reply, the 'very thin'
   needle, protect the spirit, the need for critical care,
   departing, arriving, going along, going against

3. *The Method*
   having a rule and guidance, the heavenly lights, the
   defensive qi

4. *Acupuncture: Treatment by Sun, Moon, and Planets*
   the defensive qi, to regulate, to drain, to reinforce, to 'fall
   into favour', failure in this brings illness, the importance of
   the classic text, close observation, the 'minutest of changes',
   the signs

5. *He Who Observes the Minutest of Changes*
    follow the Classics, attention to your surroundings, the
    'minutest of changes'

6. *Acupuncture: Technique, Reducing and Reinforcing*
    'square' and 'round' technique, acting with the breath, the
    qi, blood, qi and spirit, moved with great care

7. *Acupuncture: What is Meant by the Spirit*
    it is difficult to describe, but obvious, it acts as a light
    personally for yourself, its source lies in the pulse

8. *Four Common Failings in Treatment*
    neglecting Yin and Yang, recklessness, not pursuing a
    diagnosis in depth, not asking around the condition

Some questions for review can be found at the end of this chapter.

1. Origins of Five Element Acupuncture

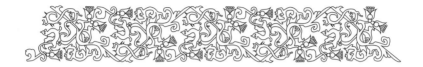

帝曰: 人生有形, 不離陰陽, 天地合氣, 別為九野, 分為四時,
月有小大, 日有短長, 萬物並至, 不可勝量, 虛實呿吟, 敢問其方.

THE YELLOW EMPEROR ASKS:

The life of the body cannot be divorced from Yin and Yang.

As the skies and earth join up their qi,

They break apart into the nine territories of the world, and divide
into the four seasons;

The months ebb and flow, the days shorten and lengthen and all
myriad creatures come into being.

We cannot count them all.

Yawning and filling up, starting to stutter and hum…

Dare I ask, is there any plan at all?

歧伯曰: 木得金而伐, 火得水而滅, 土得木而達,
金得火而缺, 水得土而絕, 萬物盡然, 不可勝竭.

Qi Bo replies:

Wood finds metal and is felled, fire meets water and is put out.

Earth finds wood and starts to grow, metal contacts fire and falls
apart, water reaches earth and is stopped;

All the myriad creatures work totally in such a manner.

You can do no better than trust to them entirely.

Zhang Jiebin: In applying Yin and Yang to heaven and earth, the *wuxing* are
exhaustive. In all the myriad things, there are those lesser and those greater, but

221

none escape the workings of 'the five' (*wuxing*). So then, when you understand that it lies in the way of the *wuxing* to control each other, the art of needling will be fixed upon and understood.

故鍼有懸布天下者五, 黔首共餘食, 莫知之也.

Therefore when the acupuncture needle was first picked up,
Under the hanging cloth of heaven's display, there were five rules.
But to the black-haired people it was like having too much to eat:
It was a situation they never knew.

Zhang Jiebin: The black-haired people were the simple people of the Jin.

Zhang Zhicong: 'Under the hanging cloth of heaven's display' refers to the time when first the *Needling Classic* was put together, to show to the people. The common villagers only ever had the strength to work the fields, and pay their rent and taxes. If they had any food left over, it went to feed the rest of the village. As for the art of acupuncture, it was not generally known or understood.

一曰治神, 二曰知養身, 三曰知毒藥為真, 四曰制砭石小大.
五曰知府藏血氣之診. 五法俱立, 各有所先.
今末世之刺也, 虚者實之, 滿者泄之, 此皆眾工所共知也.

The first is unity of spirit, the second is knowing how to aid the
     body.
The third is knowing the correct use of drastic herbs.
The fourth to control the use of stone probes.
The fifth is having a knowledge of how to examine the *zangfu*,
     blood and qi.
Once these five rules are in place altogether,
Each one of your actions will excel.
Now till the end of days, needling comprises just this:
When they are weak, then fill. When they are full, dispel.
This is it, in its entirety – it is what all practitioners totally
     understand.

若夫法天則地, 隨應而動, 和之者若響, 隨之者若影,
道無鬼神, 獨來獨往.

If you follow these rules given us by heaven and earth
Obey the moment and then move forward –

You create a harmony, as sound and echo...
And a following, as form and shadow...
There is no mystery here, no ghosts or spirits.
It is just simple. Simply come, simply go...

Wu Kun: Describing how the art is in itself enough to educate and transform the practitioner. There is no need to further employ the services of ghosts and spirits.

Zhang Jiebin: I see it in my mind and act. Then the effect will be just like magic. But this magic is my own, just the magic of my own way. It has nothing to do with ghosts or spirits. Since there are no ghosts or spirits, I simply come and go. What else could it be, anyway! In brief, Zhuangzi says, 'Simply come, simply go, this means to simply be.' In general just this is the truth of needling.

帝曰: 願聞其道. 歧伯曰:
凡刺之真, 必先治神, 五藏已定, 九候已備, 後乃存鍼.
眾脈不見, 眾凶弗聞, 外肉相得, 無以形先, 可玩往來, 乃施於人.
人有虛實, 五虛勿近, 五實勿遠, 至其當發, 間不容瞚.

The Yellow Emperor says: Please tell me more of this method!
And Qi Bo replies: In general the truth of needling lies primarily
  in a unity of spirit.
Once the five *zang* are decided, and the nine territories sorted –
After this is done, you can pick up the needle.
Where there is no beat seen –
When there is no violence heard –
When flesh and outsides hold together –
Nothingness takes precedence over form,
You can plumb the depths of profundity,
You can benefit the people.
Some have weakness, some have fullness –
If there is great weakness, you cannot go in too slow...
If there is great fullness, you cannot pull away too fast...
As it arrives, you release it in the twinkling of an eye.

手動若務, 鍼耀而勻, 靜意視義, 觀適之變.
是謂冥冥, 莫知其形, 見其烏烏, 見其稷稷.
從見其飛, 不知其誰, 伏如橫弩, 起如發機.

Your hand action should be smooth,

The work of the needle positively sparkling…
Your spirit calm, the mind at ease –
You observe it, and the transformation happens.
These are indeed the 'minutest of changes',
And they are difficult to describe,
You see it like a dark flock of crows…
Seen falling through the sky!
You follow and watch their flight
But cannot think how they do it.
It is like just when picking up a cross-bow
You stand by to slip the catch.

Zhang Jiebin: This describes the action and form of the needle. To give an example, the 'dark flock' describes the qi arriving like a dark flock of crows. 'Seen falling' describes how the qi fills, and seems to tug at you. You 'follow and watch their flight', meaning the qi comes and goes, like a flock of birds in the sky. However, you can hardly see how it is happening. The important point is that you cannot properly fathom it. That is why the text says, 'you cannot think how they do it'.

刺虛者須其實, 刺實者須其虛. 經氣已至, 慎守勿失!
深淺在志, 遠近若一,
如臨深淵, 手如握虎, 神無營於眾物.
When needling weakness, emphasise fullness.
When needling fullness, emphasise weakness.
Once the channel qi arrives, protect it, do not lose it!
Hesitant in your heart and feelings – far and near, as one,
As if approaching a deep abyss! Like grappling with a tiger!
Your mind is not concerned with anything else.

The earliest mention of the *wuxing* ('five elements') is in the old *Shujing* or *Book of Documents* of the Shang and Zhou dynasties. But above they are first used in a medical context: 'Wood finds metal and is felled, fire meets water and is put out, earth finds wood and starts to grow, metal contacts fire and falls apart, water reaches earth and is stopped. ' The point is to see into their 'mutual exchange' 相應 *xiangying*, the true science of Yin and Yang, unconcerned with imposing a plan on people. As the text says: 'Where there is no beat seen, when there is no violence heard, when flesh and outsides hold together, nothingness takes precedence over form, you can plumb the depths of profundity, you can benefit the people. ' The strange phrase 'Nothingness takes precedence over form' emphasises a humble, open attitude on the part of the practitioner. The point is the *naturalness* of treatment – 'simply come, simply go' – using *wuxing* science as the foundation. It is imperative to have a quiet, attentive mind for the *wuxing* to operate smoothly and efficiently. As Zhang Jiebin comments: '...understand that it lies in the way of the *wuxing* to control each other, and the art of needling will be fixed upon and understood. ' This is nothing abstruse or clever. You just have to see the interaction between the differing states of the physical qi in order to be able to control them. The *Suwen* states: 'When they are weak, then fill. When they are full, dispel. ' This is to describe reinforcing 補 *bu* a weak condition, and draining 瀉 *xie* a full pathogen. Then you create a harmony between Yin and Yang. 'Simply come, simply go' means 'There is no mystery here, no ghosts or spirits'. You simply do your job. It is common sense. Zhang Jiebin explains that it is just the magic of one's own art (道 *dao*, 'way, method') that provides the best results. There is no need to evoke anything else. He states: 'I see it in my mind and then act. Then the effect will be just like magic (神 *shen*). But this is just the magic of my own way. ' Simply do the job of reducing excess or building up deficiency. There is no need for any other agency.

In this chapter we see how the Chinese looked to tug, turn, encourage and deflect the body's minutest micro-electrical charges with a metal needle. What is crucial is developing a careful and restrictive technique, in order to enhance and manipulate the body's condition – aware of the 'minutest of changes'. As Zhang Jiebin suggests, you 'cannot properly fathom it'.

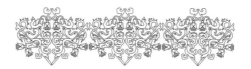

2. Opening Chapter of the *Lingshu*

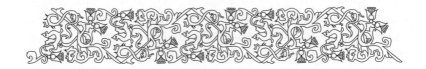

黃帝問於歧伯曰：

余子萬民，養百姓而收其租稅；余哀其不給而屬有疾病.

余欲勿使被毒藥，無用砭石，欲以微鍼通其經脈，

調其血氣，榮其逆順出入之會.

THE YELLOW EMPEROR QUESTIONED QI BO, saying:

I act as a father to the many thousands of people,

I deeply care for and feed the hundreds of families

And collect any taxes of grain from them.

I grieve when they are not provided for or when they fall ill or
   sick.

I do not want them to use drastic herbs any more, nor the stone
   piercing needles.

I want them to use the very thin needle to penetrate into the
   channels,

To regulate the qi and blood, to nourish them,

And to understand how they 'go along with or against', 'come out
   and enter in'.

令可傳於後世，必明為之法.

So from today on we should tell this to future generations.

They should understand we must construct some laws.

令終而不滅，久而不絕，易用難忘，為之經紀.

Then till the end of time, they will not be extinguished.

They will last for ever and never disappear.
We should make them practical, and difficult to forget.
And lay out their complete guiding principle.

Zhang Zhicong: The chapter heading says the 'nine needles', but the Emperor mentions a 'very thin' needle. Qi Bo says, 'the small' needle. So here, as well as the 'nine needles', we have the 'small needle'. To put it simply, the very thin needle is the small needle. Generally it is the finest of the nine needles.

歧伯答曰: 臣請推而次之, 令有綱紀, 始於一, 終於九焉.
Qi Bo replies:
As your minister, please allow me to show you and describe this.
Now I have in hand their complete guiding principle,
Beginning at one, and finishing at nine!

Zhang Jiebin: 'Beginning at one, and finishing at nine' means all factors under heaven and earth.

請言其道! 小鍼之要, 易陳而難入. 麤守形, 上守神.
Please, I will attempt to describe it!
The important point concerning the small needle
Is that it is easy to bandy about, but difficult to apply.
If you work roughly you may protect the body,
But the far better way is to protect the spirit.

Zhang Jiebin: Working roughly means protecting the visible body you see in front of you. The far better way is to protect the spirit. By far the best work is done by observing the 'minutest of changes' in spirit and qi. Not only is this true when using the needles, but in all forms of healing is this so.

神乎神, 客在門. 未睹其疾, 惡知其原?
The spirit, yes we must understand the spirit!
When the guest is at the gate,
If you cannot spy yet where the illness is lodged
How may you know its cause?

Zhang Jiebin: The spirit is the healthy qi. 'The guest' means the malign xie qi. 'The spirit, yes the spirit' means the amount of health within. You must clear up any doubt on this matter.

刺之微在速遲. 麤守關, 上守機.

Delicacy in needling rests in
Learning to work it either fast or slow.
The coarse way protects the body's joints.
The far better way is to protect its mechanisms.

Zhang Jiebin: The 'coarse way' of protecting the body's joints means protecting the fixtures of the four limbs. The 'far better way' is to protect its mechanisms (機 *ji*), which means observing the stirring qi.

機之動, 不離其空. 空中之機, 清靜而微. 其來不可逢, 其往不可追.

That impulse of the qi working rests entirely in the 'voids'.
In those spaces are its workings, clear, still and very fine.
As it arrives, you must not confront it;
At its departure, you must not rally it.

Zhang Jiebin: The 'voids' are the openings of the points. Meaning you should observe at these points, appropriately and circumspectly. As it arrives you should not confront it, because you cannot tonify what is full! As it departs you should not rally it, because you cannot drain what is empty!

知機之道者, 不可掛以發. 不知機道, 扣之不發.

If you are aware of the way the qi mechanism works,
You should not worry about or delay its expression.
If you are not aware of the way it works,
It is because it is fastened up, and not coming out.

Zhang Jiebin: If you know the way the qi mechanism works, you know there is one qi energy, and that is all. You should not worry about or delay its expression. Ultimately this means it is extremely refined and not at all in disorder. If it is 'fastened up, and not coming out', it is losing its mechanism, and the qi is not coming through.

知其往來, 要與之期.

By being aware of it arriving and departing,
You get to the crux of its timing.

麤之闇乎, 妙哉, 工獨有之.

The coarse physician is blind!

The one who sees it can marvel at it!
He alone is the one who can manage it.

Zhang Jiebin: The coarse physician is blind and unaware. The one who 'sees it can marvel at it', and alone sees what is happening.

往者為逆, 來者為順, 明知逆順, 正行無問.
Departing means you go against it,
Arriving means you go along with it.
If you are clear on both going 'along with' and 'against',
Then you can work properly with it, without questioning.

Zhang Jiebin: 'Departing' means the qi is leaving. Thus you act by going 'against it' 逆 *ni*. 'Arriving' means the qi is coming. So you act by going 'along with it' 順 *shun*.

逆而奪之, 惡得無虛? 追而濟之, 惡得無實?
To go against then is to rob from it…
How could you not cause it to weaken?
To rally it and help it out,
How could you not cause it to fill?

Zhang Jiebin: To go against the coming qi and rob from it, this is to drain (*xie*) the full condition (*shi*). How could you not cause it to weaken? To follow the leaving qi and help it out, this is to reinforce (*bu*) an empty condition (*xu*). How could you not cause it to fill?

迎之隨之, 以意和之, 鍼道畢矣.
To face up to it, to follow it –
To use your mind to resolve it,
The method of the needle is complete!

Zhang Jiebin: The method of using the needle simply means to tonify and reduce, and that is all. The methods of reduction and tonification simply mean to face up to or to follow, and that is all. You must bring about a resolution, so then the method of the acupuncture needle finds fulfilment.

Here, the Yellow Emperor sets out his aim at the opening of the *Lingshu*. He wishes to record for posterity the delicate use of the 'very thin' needle. The rough or 'coarse' physician is one who 'protects the joints': he literally identifies acupoints by using the limbs, joints and body parts. However, with the fine needle, we are instructed to look deeper. Most of the lines in this section are glossed in the next chapter but one, *Lingshu* 3. Unusually it explains again all the basic terms, that there should be no doubt. My selection is based upon that of Zhang Jiebin. As well I follow the modern LSJJS edition, which omits Huang Fumi's variant readings.

The whole of this passage demands careful study. There are varying interpretations as to the finer detail of needle manipulation, but the main drift is clear. For example: 'As it arrives, you must not confront it; at its departure, you must not rally it. ' As the qi arrives, you must not confront it; at its departure, you must not rally it. One explanation could be (although Zhang Jiebin has a different take): the situation is delicate – if the health of the patient is compromised, or else their health is just returning, do not go in too fast, or confront. On the other hand, if the malign *xie* qi is on the way out, do not act further. To do so would possibly cause it to rally and return to strength. But there is more to it than that. Note the lines stress that if the qi is 'departing', it will be empty and small. As it is small, you can go against it. This implies 'draining' or 'robbing' a full condition. When it is 'arriving' it will be in a balanced state. As it is balanced, you can go along with it. This implies 'rallying' or 'helping' an empty or weak condition. See the lines immediately following. What is evident, at least, is that watching for the 'minutest of changes' is crucial in making a good acupuncturist. We must be acutely aware of the vitality or qi of the patient – to be able to understand the timing of the needle. As Zhang Jiebin makes clear, 'The far better way is to protect the mechanisms, which means observing the stirring qi. '

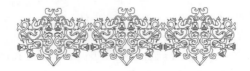

3. The Method

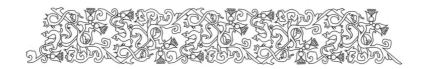

黃帝問曰: 用鍼之服, 必有法則焉, 今何法何則.

歧伯對曰: 法天則地, 合以天光.

凡刺之法, 必候日月星辰四時八正之氣, 氣定, 乃刺之.

THE YELLOW EMPEROR ASKED HIS ADVISOR:

In the service of the needle, there must be some rule or guidance.

   Could you tell me what it is? Qi Bo replied:

Our rule is in the heavens,

Guidance lies on the earth.

We model ourselves on the 'heavenly lights'.

The rule when needling must be to watch for the movement and
   qi of the sun and moon,

The stars and planets, hours and four seasons,

The eight proper sections of the year –

And when the qi has settled, at that moment to enter the needle.

是故天溫日明, 則人血淖液, 而衛氣浮, 故血易寫, 氣易行.

天寒日陰, 則人血凝泣, 而衛氣沈.

And so, when the weather is warm and the day bright,

Man's blood flows along gently, the defensive qi is floating –

So the blood easily attunes and the qi easily circulates.

When the weather is cold and the day is dull,

Man's blood congeals and the defensive qi will sink down.

In these few sections on needling methods I have included practically the whole of *Suwen* 26, the only chapter to describe in detail treatment with a fine needle. This text gives a vivid description of acupuncture protocol, as practised over 2000 years ago. Its title, 'The Eight Proper Sections and a Clear Mind', refers to how the qi of the eight 'proper sections' 正 *zheng* of the year impinges on the human body – and how needling properly involves combining 'a clear mind' (*shenming*) with a knowledge of the facts. Most contemporary editors gloss *zheng* as 正氣候 *zheng qihou* or 'proper weather', but the implication is greater. Accordingly, if we are tied to the rhythm of the seasons and cycles of the sun (year) and moon (month), and watching the weather – then our needling will be correct. The 'eight proper sections' illustrate the idea of place, space and direction. Compare the discussion on qi atmospheres coming from differing directions in Chapter V, 'The *Zangfu* and *Wuxing*'. The eight 'proper weathers' come from the eight 'proper directions' – east, south, west, north, southeast, southwest, northeast and northwest. This also suggests the solstices, equinoxes (quarter-days) and cross-quarter days of the old northern European (Celtic) calendar, Midsummer, Lammas, Michaelmas and so on. However, in China they retained a direct link to winds and climate. Again, in reproducing *Suwen* 26, I have followed the modern SWYS edition. Huang Fumi has some differences.

4. Acupuncture: Treatment by Sun, Moon and Planets

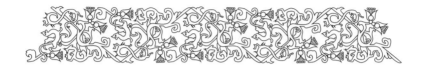

月始生, 則血氣始精, 衛氣始行. 月郭滿, 則血氣實, 肌肉堅.
月郭空, 則肌肉減, 經絡虛, 衛氣去, 形獨居.

AND AS THE MOON IS FIRST BORN so the blood and qi
    begin to clear,
And the defensive qi to circulate.
While as the moon's disc fills up, so the blood and qi solidify, and
    the muscles and flesh firm up.
As the moon's disc empties, so the muscles and flesh slacken off,
The Jingluo empty out, the defensive qi escapes,
And the form of the body is left there, alone.

是以因天時而調血氣也.
是以天寒無刺, 天溫無疑. 月生無寫, 月滿無補,
月郭空無治, 是謂得時而調之.

Therefore taking into account the timing of the skies, you regulate
    the qi and blood.
So if the weather is cold do not needle,
If the weather is warm do not moxa.
When the moon is just new do not drain,
When the moon is full do not reinforce,
When the moon's disc is empty do not treat.
This is what is meant by 'to fall into favour and treat them'.

因天之序, 盛虛之時. 移光定位, 正立而待之.

Follow the order of the skies, the timing of the weak and full.

Take your position by the shifting lights –

Stand correctly and await them.

故曰: 月生而寫, 是謂藏虛.

月滿而補, 血氣揚溢, 絡有留血, 命曰重實.

So it is said: if you drain as the moon is first born,

It means the *zang* are weakened.

If you reinforce when the moon is full,

The blood and qi become over-full, and the *luo* channels retain a
    'lingering blood'.

This the world knows as the 'doubly full'.

月郭空而治, 是謂亂經.

陰陽相錯, 真邪不別.

沈以留止, 外虛內亂, 淫邪乃起.

If the moon is empty and you treat,

It means the channels are put into disarray.

Yin and Yang are put out – and the true and malign
    indistinguishable.

They are deeply held back and blocked up,

Weak outside, and in disarray within,

And the wicked malign *xie* begins to arise.

A natural correspondence between the skies and humankind was axiomatic to the Chinese. The corollary that 'all nature and people are one' was central to their traditional science. The simplest expression of this rule in medical practice is: 'Follow the way of nature and you flourish – go against nature and you perish. ' The popular saying 'Fall into favour and treat' 得時而調之 *de shier tiao zhi* literally reads: 'Gain the time and regulate it. ' It implies using each single opportunity, every moment, to work to the best advantage of the situation.

THE RESONANCE OF SKY AND EARTH

in the sky	on earth
the moon first born	blood and qi begin to clear and the defensive qi circulates
the moon's disc fills up	blood and qi solidify, the muscles and flesh firm up
the moon's disc empties	muscles and flesh slacken, the Jingluo empty out, the defensive qi escapes
the weather cold	do not needle
the weather warm	do not moxa
the moon just new	do not drain
the moon is full	do not reinforce
the moon's disc empties	do not treat

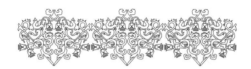

5. He Who Observes
the Minutest of Changes

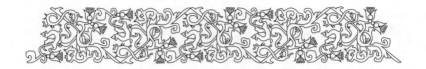

法往古者, 先知鍼經也.
驗於來今者, 先知日之寒溫, 月之虛盛.
以候氣之浮沈, 而調之於身. 觀其立有驗也.

THE PRIMARY RULE IN FOLLOWING THE ANCIENTS
Is to know and understand the *Needling Classic*.
Pay special attention to your immediate surroundings,
But first understand the warmth and cold of the day,
The ebbing and filling of the stages of the moon.
Then you can watch the rise and fall in the weather,
And bring gentle harmony to the whole person.
Closely observe where it is you stand and have proof.

觀其冥冥者, 言形氣榮衛之不形於外, 而工獨知之.
以日之寒溫, 月之虛盛, 四時氣之浮沈, 參伍相合而調之.

He who observes the minutest of changes!
This describes how the form of the qi,
Of the nutrient and defensive qi of the body
Is not shown on the outside –
But the physician on his own, he knows them both.
He takes the warmth and cold of the day,
The ebbing and filling of the shape of the moon,
The rise and fall of the four seasons,
And contrasts and combines them together into a great harmony.

工常先見之. 然而不形於外. 故曰觀於冥冥焉.

The practitioner always looks to these signs first.

He looks at how they work – not at the outward form.

This describes him who 'observes the minutest of changes'.

These last two sections describe the acute sensitivity needed when using the needle. Much is demanded of the practitioner, most especially an intimacy with seasonal and monthly change, as well as the weather. This passage attests to a natural correspondence between all living things. For the Taoist it was not just ourselves that were alive, but the whole universe as well – and why not? Why should the sun, moon, stars, rocks and clouds, trees and seas not share life with us, and be just as involved in the transforming qi as animals and plants? And to be most effective in our needling we have to be aware of them all. It is this which demands the utmost alertness and sensitivity. A few lines further on, *Suwen* 26 explains the phrase the 'minutest of changes': '…you are looking, but beyond form; you are sensing the senseless (lit. "beyond taste"); this is what is meant by the "minutest of changes" 冥冥 *mingming*, something like magic 神 *shen*, as if there, as if not. ' The implication of 'contrast and combine' 參伍 *canwu* has been discussed earlier.

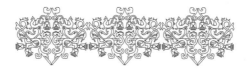

6. Acupuncture: Technique, Reducing and Reinforcing

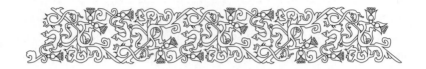

寫必用方. 方者, 以氣方盛也, 以月方滿也, 以日方溫也, 以身方定也.
WHEN REDUCING, USE THE SQUARE WAY.
'Square' means to take the qi just as it is full, the moon just filled,
The sun just at it is warming, the body just as it becomes settled.

以息方吸而內鍼, 乃復候其方吸而轉鍼, 乃復候其方呼而徐引鍼.
You go with the breath as it moves in – and enter the needle.
Then you watch until they breathe in again – and turn the needle.
Then you watch until they breathe out again – and slowly remove
    the needle.

故曰寫必用方, 其氣而行焉.
This is what is meant by 'reducing, use the square way'.
It describes how the qi is moved on.

補必用員. 員者, 行也. 行者, 移也.
When reinforcing, use the 'round' way.
'Round' means to move on. To move on means to shift.

刺必中其榮, 復以吸排鍼也.
When you needle, make sure you enter into the nutritive layer.
Next, as they breathe in, you push the qi on with the needle.

故員與方, 非鍼也. 故養神者, 必知形之肥瘦, 榮衛血氣之盛衰.

Therefore 'square' and 'round' have nothing to do with the needle.

Because when nourishing the spirit, you must understand the
    patient's physical make-up –

Whether they are fleshy or thin.

Look to the nutritive and defensive, the qi and blood,

And understand how they are filling and weakening at any one
    moment.

血氣者, 人之神. 不可不謹養.

The blood and qi make up the spirit in man.

You must always take great care with them in nourishment.

These passages are consecutive in *Suwen* 26. When using a needle
to reduce, use the 'square' way; when using a needle to reinforce,
use the 'round' way. But 'round' and 'square' should not be taken
literally. In other words, 'square' and 'round' do not identify any
fixed technique. Although we should take great care to follow
the above indications when needling, 'square' and 'round' simply
imply Yin and Yang. They impel us to take good care in each
case – they are not to do with the 'technique' of needling. When
nourishing the spirit, understand the physical make-up – whether
they are fleshy or thin, over-fed or out of condition, and so on,
whether the symptomology indicates a condition which is *shi* full
or *xu* empty, flourishing or in decline, and so on. This is to know
how to wield the needle.

Interestingly (although confusingly) in a similar section of the
Lingshu when discussing needling, the terms 'round' and 'square'
are reversed. It says that in reinforcing you act 'square' and in
reducing you act 'round'! The point – as the above last section
makes out – is that, as in so much of Chinese medicine, you need
to be clear in your method. Needling comprises both reducing
and reinforcing, Yin and Yang, both 'round' and 'square', and
your intent must be clear. I am including the *Lingshu* passages
below, as in each case they give one idea of what happens, but it
really needs personal instruction:

When reducing, use the 'round' way. Come in close to the site of the problem and twirl the needle. The qi will then move on. Quickly follow it, and then slowly take out the needle – the malign *xie* will also come out. Straighten up the needle to receive it and then shake to enlarge the hole, and the qi will move out and also speed on. When reinforcing, use the 'square' way. Guide the qi out to the skin. Now meet it at the hole, letting the left hand act as pivot, whilst the right pushes on the skin – very gently it whirls up at you and you slowly push on the needle. You must be precisely correct in this, at peace in yourself and quiet. Strong in heart and without distraction. If you want to, slightly retain the needle; when the qi arrives quickly take it out – push on the skin. If you cover over the hole on the outside, the true qi is retained. The key, when applying the needle, is never to squander the spirit.

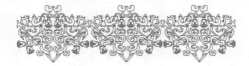

7. Acupuncture: What is Meant by the Spirit

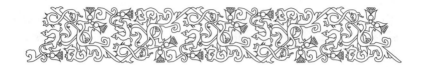

帝曰: 何謂神. 歧伯曰: 請言神.

神乎神, 耳不聞, 目明心開, 而志先, 慧然獨悟, 口弗能言, 俱視獨見.

THE YELLOW EMPEROR ASKED: And what is meant by the 'spirit'?

Qi Bo replies: Please, I will try and explain the spirit.

The spirit is the spirit,

Your senses cannot hear it.

But when the eyes are bright and the heart opened,

Then your feelings come forward, quick and alert, and you are aware of it.

But you alone understand. You cannot talk about it.

Everyone looks for it, but only you see.

適若昏, 昭然獨明. 若風吹雲. 故曰神.

三部九候為之原, 九鍼之論, 不必存也.

Suddenly, from being in the dark, there comes a light.

But it is a light for you, independently.

It is like when the wind blows away the clouds.

That is what we call the 'spirit'.

Consider the pulse, its three divisions and nine climates,

And you will find the source therein.

Then the *Canon of the Nine Needles* need not detain you further.

The three divisions describe the three lateral divisions of the pulse, along the arm. The nine climates encompass the eight directions, adding in the centre. *The Canon of the Nine Needles* was probably an earlier version of the *Lingshu*. The whole of *Suwen* 26 – the chapter describing the division of the year into eight sections, perceived with 'a clear mind' – is about the need for being sensitive with the needle. At the conclusion of the Confucian *Doctrine of the Mean*, Confucious ponders a poem from the Zhou dynasty collection, the *Book of Songs*: 'They mention that "the workings of highest Heaven are without sound, or smell". This is it exactly. ' Perhaps if we attain to the finest needling, along with the 'minutest of changes', we may aspire to such heights.

8. Four Common Failings in Treatment

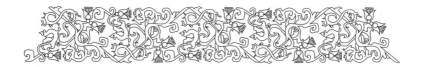

診不知陰陽逆從之理, 此治之一失矣.

IN MANAGING A DIAGNOSIS, if you do not know the first
    principles of Yin and Yang, or of following or facing the qi.

This is the first failing in treatment.

受師不卒, 妄作雜術, 謬言為道, 更名自功.
妄用砭石, 後遺身咎, 此治之二失也.

You hear the teacher, but do not complete your studies.

Then suddenly you cobble together some skill,

Using some strange terms to describe your method

And, moreover, calling it your own work.

Recklessly you use the needle, which results in an injury to the
    patient.

This is the second failing in treatment.

不適貧富貴賤之居, 坐之薄厚, 形之寒溫, 不適飲食之宜,
不別人之勇怯, 不知比類.
足以自亂, 不足以自明, 此治之三失也.

You do not succeed in finding out the wealth or poverty of their
    position,

Whether their standing has been strong or weak,

How their body responds to the temperature of the day,

And whether they are in control of their diet;

You cannot separate out whether they are brave or timid inside,
And do not know with what to compare them.
This is enough to tip you into confusion,
As you have not enough to understand the condition.
This is the third failing in treatment.

診病不問其始, 憂患飲食之失節, 起居之過度, 或傷於毒.
不先言此, 卒持寸口, 何病能中?
妄言作名, 為粗所窮, 此治之四失也.

In making the diagnosis, if you do not question its beginning,
As to whether their appetite or attitude to food has altered, or
    lifestyle changed,
Or perhaps a drastic medicine has injured them.
If you do not first ask these questions, but grab at the pulse,
Then how can you understand the disease?
You wildly make up some name for it,
Which is coarse workmanship, to the extreme.
This is the fourth failing in treatment.

These passages make it clear that the very best in medicine
depends upon seeing the patient as a whole and the power and
sensitivity of the practitioner. Xue Shengbai gives an indication
that this involves a commitment to developing an inner spirit, in
his comment on the previous chapter: 'While our practice will
derive from adapting to circumstances, subtlety comes from our
own heart and understanding. '

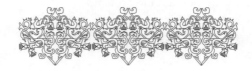

Questions for Review of Chapter VIII

1. Zhang Jiebin uses the image 'a flock of birds in the sky'. Explain *in as much detail as possible* how this could be applied to one's experience when using acupuncture.

2. Explain what is meant by 'facing up' or 'following' when needling.

3. Why do we need to follow the 'rule in the heavens' and 'guidance on the earth' when needling? Expand on this.

4. How does the moon affect the 'how and why' of needling? What have the 'minutest of changes' got to do with it?

5. Outline briefly how you understand 'reducing' and 'reinforcing'. (*Note*: There is no completely definite answer here; the question is simply giving you a chance to demonstrate that you are pursuing this subject in some depth.)

6. Describe the most common failings that occur when using the acupuncture needle.

Characters in Chapter VIII

mutual exchange 相应 *xiangying*
reinforcing a weak condition 補 *bu*
draining a full condition, expel 瀉 *xie*
one's own art, way, method 道 *dao*
magic, spirit 神 *shen*
mechanisms, workings, trigger 機 *ji*
going against 逆 *ni*
going along with 順 *shun*
eight proper sections 正 *zheng*
proper weather 正氣候 *zheng qihou*
fall into favour and treat 得時而調之 *de shier tiao zhi*
the minutest of changes, unfathomable 冥冥 *mingming*
contrast and combine 參伍 *canwu*

IX

Pathology

Man has sickness just as a tree has grubs – and sickness has its own pathology, just as grubs have a place they make their own.

Key Ideas

1. *A Typology of Conditions*
   the pathology of wind, cold, emotion, damp, heat, fire, above and below, 'reversing', swellings, and so on

2. *Elemental, Seasonal and Dietary Injuries*
   cold, summer heat, damp, seasonal injuries, dietary excess, symptomology

3. *Elemental Forms and Body Isomorphism*
   build and character, wood, fire, earth, metal and water people, their tendency

4. *A Complete Explanation of the Full or Weak*
   the malign *xie*, fullness 'stolen away', weakness, general therapeutics

5. *Cold and Heat, Yin and Yang, Inner and Outer*
   Yin and Yang mechanisms, outer, inner, cold and heat pathologies, symptomology

6. *The Five Full, the Five Weak*
   the pulse in extremis, symptomology, survival

7. *On the Temperament*
   temperament and qi, the nutrient and defensive qi, the *sanjiao*, cold, excitement, fear, worry, tiredness

8. *How Heat Represents in the Face*
   fever and its progression

9. *On the Progression of Fevers*
   fever, Yangming, Shaoyang, Taiyin and Shaoyin stages

10. *On Various Kinds of Pain*
    the circulation, cold, pain typology, weakening, sluggishness

11. *On Bi Immobility Syndromes*
    bi immobility, wind, cold, damp, *zang* conditions, pain, numbness, sweating

12. *On Dreaming 1*
    dreams, weakness in the *zang*

13. *On Dreaming 2*
    dreaming, full conditions, lodged conditions

14. *Times of Dying: Channel Collapse*
    collapse of the Yin channels, five Yin, five Yang, timing the collapse, *wuxing* science

15. *Times of Dying: Seasonal Collapse*
    seasonal collapse, winter, spring, summer, autumn, Yin and Yang

16. *The Collapse of the Channels*
    channel collapse, Yin and Yang typology, death signs

Some questions for review can be found at the end of this chapter.

1. A Typology of Conditions

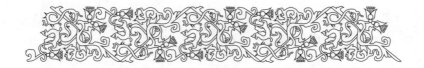

諸風掉眩, 皆屬於肝, 諸寒收引, 皆屬於腎, 諸氣膹鬱, 皆屬於肺,
諸濕腫滿, 皆屬於脾, 諸熱瞀瘛, 皆屬於火, 諸痛癢瘡, 皆屬於心,
諸厥固泄, 皆屬於下, 諸痿喘嘔, 皆屬於上.

ALL KINDS OF WIND CONDITIONS, that lead to
   disturbance and dizziness; they belong to the liver.

All kinds of cold conditions, that make you pull in and retire;
   they belong to the kidneys.

All kinds of emotional upsets, that lead to you losing your cool
   and sluggishness; they belong to the lungs.

All kinds of damp conditions, that lead to a feeling of swelling
   and fullness; they belong to the spleen.

All kinds of heat conditions, that create confusion and
   convulsions; they belong to fire.

All kinds of painful itching and sores on the skin; they belong to
   the heart.

All kinds of 'reversing' illnesses, with either retention or
   incontinence; they belong below.

All kinds of illnesses with wasting and withering in the limbs,
   gasping or retching; they belong to above.

諸禁鼓栗, 如喪神守, 皆屬於火, 諸痙項強, 皆屬於濕,
諸逆沖上, 皆屬於火, 諸脹腹大, 皆屬於熱, 諸燥狂越, 皆屬於火.

All kinds of inhibitions, with shivering and chattering, as if you
   have lost presence of mind; they belong to fire.

All kinds of spasms, stiffness and cramps in the neck; they belong
   to the damp.

All kinds of conditions where the energy reverses its true course
and rushes on above; they belong to fire.

All kinds of conditions where the belly is swollen out and
enlarged; they belong to heat.

All kinds of conditions with impulsive or wild behaviour and
leaping about; they belong to fire.

諸暴強直, 皆屬於風, 諸病有聲, 鼓之如鼓, 皆屬於熱,
諸病胕腫, 疼酸驚駭, 皆屬於火, 諸轉反戾, 水液渾濁, 皆屬於熱,
諸病水液, 澄徹清冷, 皆屬於寒, 諸嘔吐酸, 暴注下迫, 皆屬於熱.

All kinds of conditions with fierce cramps, being stiff standing up
and unable to bend; they belong to wind.

All kinds of sicknesses that create sounds like rumbling drums;
they belong to heat.

All kinds of sicknesses with light swellings, pain and soreness, and
being startled or shook up; they belong to fire.

All kinds of conditions with twisted limbs, turned and drawn up,
Where the body fluids are dirtied and unclear; they belong to fire.

All kinds of sicknesses where the body fluids remain transparent
and clear; they belong to cold.

All kinds of conditions with retching, vomiting and the bringing
up of sour fluid,
Where there is fierce discharge or severe constipation; they belong
to heat.

This grand passage is unparalleled in giving a simple pathology, the
so-called 'nineteen conditions'. It is an overview of qi dynamics,
embracing *wuxing* ideas to help create a clearer understanding of
the world. It begins with pathologies of the liver, kidneys, lungs
and spleen, fire and the heart; and then continues with below
and above, fire, damp, heat, wind and cold. Symptoms relating
to fire predominate. All in all, a comprehensive picture of the
most common underlying conditions, tying them to an elemental
wuxing pathology.

A SIMPLE PATHOLOGY

condition	effects	belongs to
wind	disturbance, dizziness	the liver
cold	pull in, retire	the kidneys
emotional	loss of cool, sluggishness	the lungs
damp	a swelling feeling, fullness	the spleen
heat	confusion, convulsions	fire
itching and sores	sores on the skin	the heart
'reversing'	retention, incontinence	below
wasting, withering	gasping, retching	above
inhibitions	shivering, chattering, no presence of mind	fire
spasms, stiffness,	cramps in the neck	damp
energy reversing	rushing above	fire
belly swollen	enlarged	heat
impulsive behaviour	wild and leaping about	fire
fierce cramps, stiff	unable to bend	wind
sickness with sound	like rumbling drums	heat
light swellings, pain	startled, shaken up	fire
limbs twisted, or drawn up	body fluids are dirtied and unclear	fire
body fluids clear	body fluids transparent	cold
retching, bringing up sour fluid	fierce discharge or severe constipation	heat

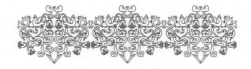

2. Elemental, Seasonal and Dietary Injuries

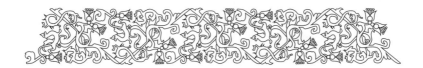

因於寒, 欲如運樞, 起居如驚, 神氣乃浮.
因於暑, 汗煩則喘喝, 靜則多言, 體若燔炭, 汗出而散.
因於濕, 首如裹, 濕熱不攘, 大筋緛短, 小筋弛長.
緛短為拘, 弛長為痿.

WHEN CAUGHT BY THE COLD,
Your desires move around like a spinning hub,
You go about your daily life as if in fear,
Your mental ideas floating.
When caught by the summer heat, you sweat.
You become anxious, so then you take quick breaths and become thirsty.
If caught and inactive, you use too many words.
Your body is like a glowing coal, your sweat escapes and disperses.
When caught by the damp, your head feels wrapped in a clothen bundle.
If the damp heat is not driven out, the larger sinews get taut and shorten,
And the smaller sinews slacken and lengthen.
Those taut and shortened go into spasm;
Those slack and lengthened become weak.

春傷於風, 邪氣留連, 乃為洞泄. 夏傷於暑, 秋為痎瘧.
秋傷於濕, 上逆而欬, 發為痿厥. 冬傷於寒, 春必溫病.

If in spring you are injured by the wind,

251

The malign qi lingers on and connects up,
And it becomes urgent diarrhoea.
If in summer you are injured by the summer heat,
In autumn it turns to an intermittent fever, coming every other
   day.
If in autumn you are injured by the damp,
It rises above, reversing its course, and turns to coughing.
It develops eventually into a wasting sickness.
If in winter you are injured by the cold,
In spring you must suffer a 'warm sickness'.

味過於酸, 肝氣以津, 脾氣乃絕.
味過于鹹, 大骨氣勞, 短肌, 心氣抑.
味過于甘, 心氣喘滿, 色黑, 腎氣不衡.
味過于苦, 脾氣不濡, 胃氣乃厚.
味過于辛, 筋脈沮弛, 精神乃央.

If the food eaten is too sour, the liver qi creates *jin* juices and the
   spleen qi collapses.
If the food eaten is too salty, the qi of the long bones wears out,
Their muscles contract and the heart's power is repressed.
If the food eaten is too sweet, the heart qi creates difficulty in
   breathing,
And a sense of fullness comes, the complexion blackens and the
   kidney qi lacks power.
If the food eaten is too bitter, the spleen qi becomes unmoistened,
   and the stomach qi over-full.
If the food eaten is too pungent, the sinews and vessels are ruined,
They lose tension and the mental strength almost gives up.

This passage discusses elemental, seasonal and dietary injuries and
their influence on bodily health. The pathologies of cold, summer
heat and damp are recorded, then their combination with season
and time of year. A heat injury in the summer turns to a fever in
the autumn. An injury from the autumn damp develops into a
wasting sickness. Injuries from a cold winter develop in spring
into a 'warm sickness'. The second part again states very clearly

how dietary excesses injure the internal *zang* organs. Too sour food injures the liver and spleen, too salty attacks the heart, too sweet goes to the heart and lungs, and eventually the kidneys, too bitter to the spleen and stomach, and too pungent attacks the sinews and mental strength. Much of this is common sense – the avoidance of pathological invasion by seasonal and dietary factors.

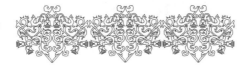

3. Elemental Forms
and Body Isomorphism

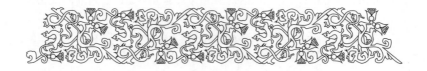

木形之人, 比于上角似於蒼, 小頭, 長面大肩背直身小, 手足好.
有才, 勞心, 少力多憂, 勞於事.
能春夏, 不能秋冬, 感而病生足厥陰, 佗佗然.

THE FORM OF WOOD PEOPLE resonates with the upper *jue* tone (pentatonic 'mi') on the scale. They are of a greenish complexion, with a small head, long face, large shoulders and back, an upright body and small hands and feet.

> If they have an ability, it is that they love to tax the mind.
> They have less strength, but are more painstaking in their affairs.

They have energy spring and summer; but none autumn or winter. When afflicted by disease through the foot Jueyin, they may become self-possessed.

火形之人, 比於上徵, 赤色廣䏚脫面小頭, 好肩背, 髀腹小手足.
行安地疾心, 行搖肩背肉滿.
有氣輕財, 少信多慮, 見事明好顏, 急心不壽暴死.
能春夏, 不能秋冬, 秋冬感而病生, 手少陰核核.

THE FORM OF FIRE PEOPLE resonates with the upper *zhi* tone (pentatonic 'soh') on the scale. They are red in complexion, with broad muscles on the back, a keen face, small head, good shoulders, thighs, back and belly, and small hands and feet.

254

When they get involved, they feel things strongly.
They can get agitated, with body, shoulders and back all
   involved.
They have strong feelings, but slight ability.
Small trust, many ideas.
They see matters clearly, put a good face on things and have a
   quick mind –
But do not live long and can die suddenly.

They have energy spring and summer, but none autumn or winter.
Autumn and winter, when afflicted by disease through the hand
Shaoyin, they may become over-bound up in things.

土形之人, 比於上宮, 黃色圓面,
大頭美肩背, 大腹, 美股脛, 小手足, 多肉, 上下相稱行安地.
舉足浮, 安心, 好利人不喜權勢, 善附人也.
能秋冬, 不能春夏, 春夏感而病生, 足太陰, 敦敦然.

THE FORM OF EARTH PEOPLE resonates with the upper *gong*
tone (pentatonic 'doh') on the scale. They are yellowy in complexion,
have a round face, large head, fine thighs and calves, but small
hands and feet. They are well fleshed out, but on the whole well
proportioned.

When they get involved, they get to their feet willingly, they
   are calm.
They love to profit people, but are not good with authority.
They are good at supporting others.

They have energy autumn and winter, but none spring or summer.
Spring and summer, when afflicted by disease through the foot
Taiyin, they may become over-generous.

金形之人比於上商, 方面白色,
小頭小肩背小腹, 小手足如骨發踵外骨輕.
身清廉, 急心靜悍, 善為吏.
能秋冬, 不能春夏, 春夏感而病生, 手太陰敦敦然.

THE FORM OF METAL PEOPLE resonates with the upper *shang*
tone (pentatonic 'ray') on the scale. They look you square in the
face and have a palish complexion. They have a small head, slight

shoulders and back, small belly and small hands and feet. It is as if the bones protrude out by the heel.

> Although their bones are slight, they are incorruptible at heart,
> With a quick mind, fiercely detached, and good with
> officialdom.

Autumn and winter they have energy, but none in spring or summer. Spring and summer, when afflicted with disease in the hand Taiyin, they may become too pure in mind and exacting.

水形之人, 比於上羽, 黑色面不平,

大頭廉頤, 小肩大腹動手足.

發行搖身, 下尻長, 背延延然. 不敬畏善欺紹人, 戮死.

能秋冬, 不能春夏, 春夏感而病生, 足少陰汗汗然.

THE FORM OF WATER PEOPLE resonates with the upper *yu* tone (pentatonic 'lah') on the scale. People such as this are of a dark complexion. Their faces are marked or well creased. They have a large head and broad chins, small shoulders, a large belly and restless hands and feet.

> When they act it agitates the whole body.
> They are long in the tailbone, with a long back.
> They are not respectful of others and good at winding people
> up.
> Their death can be violent.

Autumn and winter they have energy, but none spring or summer. Spring and summer, when afflicted with disease through the foot Shaoyin, they may fall foul of events and suffer ruin.

This gives the famous typology of the five characters of people – wood, fire, earth, metal and water. The text is from *Lingshu* 64. Because of the importance of this chapter (it is the earliest attachment of 'elements' to 'person'), I have carefully looked at two surviving versions: that in the *Lingshu* and also that recorded in Huang Fumi's *ABC of Acupuncture and Moxibustion* (*Zhenjiu Jiayi Jing*). There are considerable differences – but I have chosen to stay with the *Lingshu*, probably the earliest. The only change I make is to omit the redundant seven characters in each section which attach 'element' (*xing*) to sound. There is considerable variation, but the broad sweep is the same. Several passages have fallen out and characters 'morphed' – possibly due to copying errors.

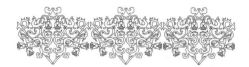

FIVE ELEMENTAL FORMS OF PEOPLE

human form	wood	fire	earth	metal	water
resonating tone	jue (mi)	zheng (soh)	gong (doh)	shang (ray)	yu (lah)
complexion	greenish	red	yellowy	palish	dark
bodily appearance	a small head, long face, large shoulders and back, an upright body and small hands and feet	broad back muscles, a keen face, small head, good shoulders, thighs, back and belly, and small hands and feet	a round face, large head, fine thighs and calves, small hands and feet, well proportioned	a small head, slight shoulders and back, small belly, hands and feet	marked or well-creased face, a large head, broad chin, small shoulders, a large belly and restless hands and feet
strengths	they love to tax the mind	they feel strongly, can get agitated but have slight ability	they get to their feet willingly and are calm	incorruptible at heart	their actions agitate the whole body, they are long in the tailbone and back
character	have less strength but are more painstaking in their affairs	have slight ability, small trust, but many ideas, see clearly and have a quick mind, but can die suddenly	love to profit people, but are not good with authority	with a quick mind, fiercely detached and good with officialdom	not respectful of others and good at winding people up, their death can be violent
have energy	spring and summer	spring and summer	autumn and winter	autumn and winter	autumn and winter
have no energy	autumn and winter	autumn and winter	spring and summer	spring and summer	spring and summer
afflicted through	Liver foot Jueyin	Heart hand Shaoyin	Spleen foot Taiyin	Lung hand Taiyin	Kidney foot Shaoyin
resulting disease	may become self-possessed	over-bound up in things	may become over-generous	may become too pure in mind and exacting	may fall foul of events and suffer ruin

4. A Complete Explanation of the Full or Weak

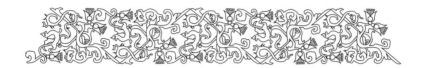

邪氣盛則實, 精氣奪則虛.

IF THE MALIGN QI IS ABUNDANT, it means fullness.
If the essential qi has been stolen, it means weakness.

Li Zhongzi: These two sentences form the guiding principle for the medical profession. They mark the baseline for a thousand generations to come. Perhaps their words seem slight and easily understood, but their implication is truly profound and difficult to construe. So then the malign qi is the wind, cold, summer heat, damp, dryness and fire. While the essential qi means the healthy qi (*zhengqi*), namely the minutely transformed substances formed from food (*guqi*).

Li Zhongzi: Being 'abundant', it is 'full' (*shi*); meaning the malign qi is actually expanding and generally known as a 'full symptom'. If something is strong, you must expel (*xie*) it. If the condition is severe, then use sweating (diaphoretics), vomiting (emetics) or downward-acting medicines (cathartics, laxatives). If the condition is light, then clear (*qing*) the fire and subdue the qi. This is how to do it. If the qi 'has been stolen', then there is a 'weakness', due to wasted *jing* or lost blood, overusing the body or wearying the mind. These conditions are generally known as 'stolen within'. Sweating, purging below, vomiting or clearing out are generally known as 'stolen without'. A lack of courage or a dispirited mind generally indicates 'weak' symptoms. When all 'three climes' (positions of the pulse) are forceless, it is generally called a 'weak' pulse. If the condition is weak, you must tonify (*bu*). If the condition is light, then use warmth (or gentle tonics, *wen*) to tonify it. If the condition is severe, use more heat to tonify it. This is how to do it.

The above lines on full and weak conditions outline the importance of the strong or full 實 *shi* and weak or empty 虛 *xu* distinction. Once this is made, it points clearly to an appropriate therapeutic action. The six malign climatic factors are 'wind, cold, summer heat, damp, dryness and fire', also known as the 'six source qi' (六元氣 *liu yuan qi*), being transformations of the single qi, the atmosphere of the skies and its interaction with the earth.

Practitioners need to comprehend how an understanding of pathology arises during an examination. Then the actions of 'expelling' 瀉 *xie* and tonifying 補 *bu* naturally follow. Below follows the rest of Li Zhongzi's commentary on these two lines, noting the careful reasoning needed in setting both full and weak conditions to rights. The following discussion applies mainly to herbal therapeutics:

> One well versed in these rules only separates out these two characters, 'full' and 'weak', and that's all. They cover all conditions: the 'largely full', the 'largely weak'; the 'less full', the 'less weak'; the 'as if full' and the 'as if weak'. Again, value making a careful judgement. In largely weak conditions, reinforce. It is best to act swiftly, and best to use gentle tonics – if you delay there will be no result. In largely full conditions, attack. It is best to act rapidly, and best to use more potent medicines – if you are slow, their life will have departed. A less weak condition implies seven parts reinforcing and three parts attacking. Work on just one aspect of the condition. A less full condition implies seven parts attacking and three parts reinforcing. Guard against it being too severe. As for those conditions which are 'as if weak' and 'as if strong', about these the whole world is unclear. If a more weak condition shows signs of fullness, to drain instead will harbour the wrong within. While if a very strong condition has an emaciated appearance, to mistakenly reinforce will benefit the sickness. You cannot be too careful in separating these out. In healing, you must perpetually use the utmost care. Alas indeed! If the condition is strong and you mistakenly reinforce it, it

positively benefits the malign force – although you can go to their aid while the calamity is still small. If the condition is weak and you mistakenly attack it, the true qi is at once finished! Nobody can ever restore it and the calamity is very great. Our foremost concern must be with life and death; good and bad are indeterminate and insignificant. As arbiters of human destiny, we must take care!

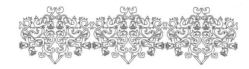

5. Cold and Heat, Yin and Yang, Inner and Outer

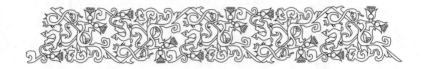

帝曰: 陽虛則外寒, 陰虛則內熱,
陽盛則外熱, 陰盛則內寒, 余已聞之矣. 不知其所由然也.
岐伯曰: 陽受氣於上焦, 以溫皮膚分肉之間, 令寒氣在外,
則上焦不通, 上焦不通, 則寒氣獨留於外, 故寒慄.

THE YELLOW EMPEROR ASKS, saying:

> If Yang is weak, the outsides remain cold.
> If Yin is weak, the insides remain hot.
> If Yang is filled, the outsides remain hot.
> If Yin is filled, the insides remain cold.
> I do not understand. How do these all come about?

Qi Bo answers: The Yang receives its qi from the upper *jiao*, to warm the skin and the spaces between the muscles. Now if the cold is outside, the upper *jiao* is not flowing freely. If the upper *jiao* is not flowing freely, cold remains, by itself, on the outside. Hence you feel cold and shiver.

Li Zhongzi: If Yang is weak there is no qi to warm the skin.

陰虛生內熱奈何?
岐伯曰: 有所勞倦, 形氣衰少, 谷氣不盛, 上焦不行, 下脘不通.
胃氣熱, 熱氣熏胸中, 故內熱.

> If Yin is weak, it generates heat inside.
> How does this come about?

Qi Bo answers: It comes about through overwork and tiredness. The physical qi is much reduced and there is improper digestion. The upper *jiao* is blocked and the lower ducts do not open freely. Then the stomach qi heats up and the heat produces stuffiness in the chest. Hence the insides remain hot.

Li Zhongzi: The Yin qi nourishes the interior. If you overwork and are tired, the stomach and spleen are injured. The spleen commands the muscles and flesh, but also the transporting and transforming of the qi obtained from food (*gu qi*) in order to produce the true qi. As the 'soil' (stomach and spleen) diminishes, so the form and central bodily qi (*zhong qi*) both decline and the qi obtained from food is slightly diminished. The spleen is weakened, the qi sinks below, the upper *jiao* becomes blocked and the lower ducts certainly do not open freely. The Yin of the spleen is insufficient, the stomach heats up. The lungs dwell in the chest and the heat rises to produce stuffiness in the lungs, so then there is heat inside. Overwork and tiredness are mentioned here as injuring the spleen and causing symptoms like those above. If it is sexual desires that have caused the damage, the 'real water' (*zhen shui*) is drained dry and the fire left without anything to fear. It becomes overbearing and punishes the metal of the lungs. This is 'inner heat' and most difficult to heal.

陽盛生外熱奈何?
岐伯曰: 上焦不通利, 則皮膚致密, 腠理閉塞, 玄府不通,
衛氣不得泄越, 故外熱.

If Yang is filled, the outsides remain hot.
How does this come about?

Qi Bo answers: If the upper *jiao* is not flowing freely, the skin closes off. The pores of the skin are stopped up and the innermost recesses of the body unreached. The defensive qi is not able to escape and run over the skin. Hence the outsides remain hot.

Li Zhongzi: The Yang commands the above, and also the exterior. If the Yang is overbearing, above is in stasis and there is heat externally. This is a sign of a 'cold injury'.

陰盛生內寒奈何?
岐伯曰: 厥氣上逆, 寒氣積於胸中而不瀉, 不瀉則溫氣去寒獨留,
則血凝泣, 凝則脈不通, 其脈盛大以濇, 故中寒.

If Yin is filled, it creates cold inside.
How does this come about?

Qi Bo answers: The weakening qi rises up above, rebelling. The cold qi accumulates within the chest and cannot clear. If it cannot clear, the warm qi departs. Then the cold alone remains and the blood congeals. As it congeals, the pulse does not come freely. The pulse becomes full and enlarged, thereby dragging. Hence there remains cold within.

Li Zhongzi: Cold qi moves into the organs and the Yang qi simply departs. The cold alone is retained and, just like all creatures at the order of winter, the qi 'hides away because of the bitter cold'. Hence the pulse does not come freely but drags. This is a sign of an internal injury.

Now we pass on to a discussion of the pathologies of cold and heat, Yin and Yang, and inner and outer, six of the so-called 'eight principles' 八綱 *ba gang*. The other two, *shi* full and *xu* empty, were discussed in the previous section. These descriptions are useful technically, to understand the pathology of disturbance within the body – especially with reference to the upper *jiao*. Li Zhongzi's commentary explains well the causes and intricacies of *yinyang* dynamics. Note the particularly aggravating features of 'inner heat', caused by long depletion of the Yin of the kidneys. For the 'outsides remaining hot', and 'cold injury' 傷寒 *shanghan*, see Section 9.

6. The Five Full,
the Five Weak

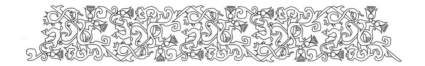

帝曰: 願聞五實五虛? 岐伯曰:
脈盛, 皮熱, 腹脹, 前後不通, 悶瞀, 此謂五實.
脈細, 皮寒, 氣少, 泄利前後, 飲食不入, 此謂五虛.
帝曰: 其時有生者何也? 岐伯曰:
漿粥入胃, 泄注止, 則虛者活, 身汗得後利, 則實者活. 此其候也.

THE YELLOW EMPEROR ASKS, saying: But what is it I hear about the 'five full' and 'five weak'?

Qi Bo answers, saying: The pulse filled, the skin hot, the belly swollen, neither convenience moving freely, the eyes glazing over. These are the 'five full'. The pulse thready, the skin cold, the energy very little, diarrhoea or incontinence, and unable to keep food or liquid down. These are the 'five weak'.

The Yellow Emperor replies: But sometimes people survive. Why is that?

Qi Bo answers: With some, when rice gruel is eaten, the diarrhoea and dissipation may halt. So then, even when weak you may survive. If the whole body breaks into a sweat and you are able to move your bowels, even when the condition is full you may survive. This is what I have seen.

Li Zhongzi: Both the 'five full' and 'five weak' are fatal signs.

Xue Shengbai: Both the 'five full' or 'five weak' together are fatal. Obviously, if your qi is weak it will ultimately finish, and when it finishes you die. In principle this must be so, so if you have 'five full', why is this also fatal? In general for the evil to find some place to invade, your qi must have been weakened. If you do not let it slip away, you will not die. So then, this is merely the same as your qi finishing. However, both full and weak conditions have true and false presentations. It is these which you should separate out most carefully!

This passage outlines two particularly severe conditions. Full conditions include a hot skin, swollen abdomen, blockages in moving the bowel or passing urine, and losing sensibility. Empty conditions include a thready pulse, a cold skin, little energy, diarrhoea or incontinence, and being unable to keep food or drink down. Li Zhongzi notes that 'both five full and five weak are fatal signs'. Xue Shengbai explains how both the 'five full' and 'five weak' depend ultimately on a weakened body. However, the text also illustrates how, even in extreme cases, a little light food, encouraging sweating or moving the bowels, can bring remission and improvement.

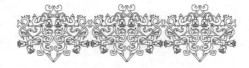

7. On the Temperament

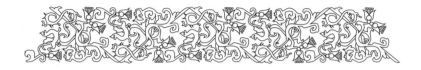

帝曰: 余知百病生於氣也.
怒則氣上, 喜則氣緩, 悲則氣消, 恐則氣下, 寒則氣收,
炅則氣泄, 驚則氣亂, 勞則氣耗, 思則氣結.
九氣不同, 何病之生?

THE YELLOW EMPEROR SAYS: I know that all sickness is created by the temperament.

> When you are angry, the qi is rising.
> When you are happy, it slows down.
> When you are sorrowful, it is vanishing.
> When you are fearful, it falls below.
> When you are cold, it contracts.
> When you are hot, it is dissipating.
> When you are frightened, it is in turmoil.
> As you get tired, it becomes wasted.
> When you worry, it gets tied in knots.

These nine temperaments are not all similar. So how is it that they create sickness?

岐伯曰: 怒則氣逆, 甚則嘔血及飧泄, 故氣上矣.
喜則氣和志達, 榮衛通利, 故氣緩矣.

Qi Bo replies, saying: When you are angry, the qi acts contrary to its usual course. In extreme cases you vomit blood, or there is diarrhoea with undigested food. This is surely because your qi rises.

When you are happy, the qi is peaceful and the will fulfilled. Both the nutrient and defensive qi are now flowing freely and well. This is surely because your qi is slowing down.

悲則心系急, 肺布葉舉, 而上焦不通, 榮衛不散, 熱氣在中, 故氣消矣.
恐則精卻, 卻則上焦閉, 閉則氣還, 還則下焦脹, 故氣不行矣.

When you are sorrowful, the heart system is in an acute state. The lungs spread out, raising up their separate lobes, and the upper *jiao* is prevented from flowing freely. The nutrient and defensive qi cannot be dispersed, and the heated qi stays within. This is surely because your qi is vanishing.

When you are fearful, your *jing* is cut back. As it is cut back so the upper *jiao* closes off. As it closes off, the qi turns back. As it turns back below, the lower *jiao* swells out. This is surely because your qi is not circulating.

寒則腠理閉, 氣不行, 故氣收矣.
炅則腠理開, 榮衛通, 汗大泄, 故氣泄.
驚則心無所依, 神無所歸, 慮無所定, 故氣亂矣.

When you are cold, the pores of the skin close off. The qi is not circulating. This is surely because the qi contracts.

When you are excited, the pores of the skin open. The nutrient and defensive qi flow out freely and the sweat streams out. This is surely because the qi is dissipating.

When you are frightened, the heart has nothing to support it. Your mind has no place to return to. You feel anxious and uncertain. This is surely because the qi is in turmoil.

勞則喘息汗出, 外內皆越, 故氣耗矣.
思則心有所存, 神有所歸, 正氣留而不行, 故氣結矣.

When you get tired, there is difficulty in breathing and you perspire. Both inner and outer are encroached upon. This is surely because the qi is wasted.

When you are worried, the heart is holding something back. Your mind has something it keeps returning to. The healthy qi stagnates and cannot be expressed. This is surely because the qi gets tie knots.

This section on the 'temperament' 氣 *qi* explains clearly how differing medical conditions are created through differing temperaments. The qi moves in a multitude of ways: during anger, happiness, sorrow and fearful states, when cold or heated, when frightened, or during tiredness. These temperaments are not all the same – and neither are their qi. The section illustrates nicely how the actual physical state of the qi determines the mode of disease. Compare my note on the emotions in Chapter V, Section 4. This explains how Chinese medicine – going directly to the physical cause – can be so effective for mental or emotional problems. In this passage Huang Fumi's text varies in some minor ways.

QI STRATA

the condition	the qi
angry	is rising
happy	slows down
sorrowful	is vanishing
fearful	falls below
feel cold	contracts
feel hot	is dissipating
frightened	is in turmoil
get tired	becomes wasted
worry	gets tied in knots

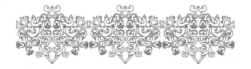

8. How Heat Represents in the Face

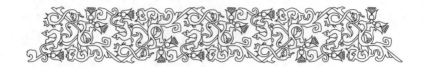

肝熱病者, 左頰先赤, 心熱病者, 顏先赤, 脾熱病者, 鼻先赤,
肺熱病者, 右頰先赤, 腎熱病, 頤先赤.

IF THE LIVER HAS HEAT, the left cheek first reddens.
If the heart has heat, the forehead first reddens.
If the spleen has heat, the nose first reddens.
If the lungs have heat, the right cheek first reddens.
If the kidneys have heat, the chin first reddens.

Li Zhongzi: The liver corresponds to the east, so the left cheek first reddens. The heart corresponds to the south, so the forehead first reddens. The spleen corresponds to the central region, so the nose first reddens. The lungs correspond to the west, so the right cheek first reddens. The kidneys correspond to the north, so the chin first reddens.

This shows a simple schema using the differential of the five *zang* organs to represent heat (usually the first flushing of fever) on the face. The associated directions (left, right, above, below – see Chapter V, Sections 3 and 4) are used to diagnose which *zang* organ is at fault.

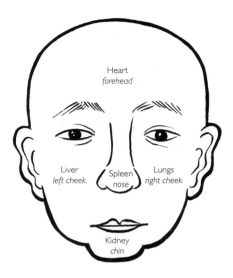

The appearance of redness in the face due to fever

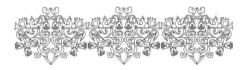

9. On the Progression of Fevers

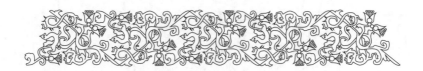

黄帝問曰：今夫熱病者，皆傷寒之類也，或愈或死，
其死皆以六七日之間，其愈皆以十日以上者，何也.

THE YELLOW EMPEROR ASKS, saying: Now as to fevers, I mean
the kind caused by a cold injury. In some cases you recover, and in
some cases you die. When death takes place it is usually over a six
or seven-day period. When you recover it is usually after ten days or
more. Now why is this?

歧伯對曰：巨陽者，諸陽之屬也.
其脈連於風府，故為諸陽主氣也，人之傷於寒也，則為病熱，熱雖甚不死.
其兩感於寒而病者，必不免於死.

Qi Bo replies: It concerns the chief Yang channel which connects up
with the several other Yang channels.

> This vessel joins up with them at the 'palace of the winds'.
> Hence it aids the several Yang in command of their qi.
> When someone is injured by the cold and it turns into a fever,
> Even though the fever is extreme it will not necessarily be
>   fatal.
> But if two channels are caught by the cold and fall sick, you
>   will be lucky to escape death.

傷寒一日，巨陽受之，故頭項痛，腰脊強.
二日陽明受之，陽明主肉，其脈俠鼻，絡於目.
故身熱目痛而鼻乾，不得臥也.

The first day the chief Yang receives a cold injury, so the head and neck ache and the waist and back stiffen. The second day the Yangming receives it. The Yangming is in command of the flesh. Its vessel passes close by the sides of the nose to link up with the eyes. So then the body becomes feverish, the eyes ache and the nose feels dry. You are unable to sleep.

三日少陽受之, 少陽主膽, 其脈循脅絡於耳, 故胸脅痛而耳聾.
三陽經絡, 皆受其病, 而未入於臟者, 故可汗而已.
四日太陰受之太陰脈布胃中, 絡於嗌, 故腹滿而溢乾.

The third day the Shaoyang receives it. The Shaoyang is in command of the gallbladder. Its vessel follows the ribs to link up with the ear, so the chest and ribs ache and you become deaf.

The three Yang channels and sub-channels all having received the sickness, it has not yet entered the *zang* organs. So it should be sweated out and ended.

Then the fourth day the Taiyin receives it. The Taiyin vessel spreads into the stomach and is connected to the back of the throat, so the belly feels full and the throat dry.

五日少陰受之. 少陰脈貫腎, 絡於肺, 系舌本, 故口燥舌乾而渴.
六日厥陰受之. 厥陰脈循陰器而絡於肝, 故煩滿而囊縮.

The fifth day the Shaoyin receives it. The Shaoyin vessel passes through the kidneys, connects up to the lungs, and ties up at the root of the tongue. So then the mouth is parched, the tongue dry and you feel thirsty.

The sixth day the Jueyin receives it. The Jueyin vessel follows the sex organs and connects up with the liver, so then you feel anxious, with a feeling of fullness, and the scrotum shrivels.

三陰三陽, 五臟六腑皆受病, 榮衛不行, 五臟不通, 則死矣.
其未滿三日者, 可汗而已, 其滿三日者, 可泄而已.

Once the three Yin and three Yang, five *zang* and six *fu* have all received the sickness, the nutrient and defensive qi is prevented from circulating and the five *zang* from communicating, so the sickness will be fatal indeed!

winds

If it has not yet reached its peak by the third day, one should sweat it out and end it. If it has reached its peak by the third day, one should purge it out and end it.

From the chapter on 'fevers', *Suwen* 31. The next three sections describe the occurrence of fever, pain and *bi* immobility syndromes, due to the invasion of malign factors. Collectively they give examples of *yinyang* and *wuxing* reasoning applied to the five *zang* organs and as an aid in explaining the mechanism of any medical condition. Fever comes about through a 'cold injury' and through cold invading the body – which then turns to heat, passing through into the channels. Pain involves blocking, also mainly caused by the cold; and *bi* immobility may involve either heat, cold or damp obstructing the channels.

The above section discusses the progression of the fever through the Yang and then Yin channels. The question is, why are some fevers fatal, and others not? The answer is that, even though the fever is full, if it does not progress through the channels the patient will recover, even if it takes a little longer. If it progresses from the 'chief' Yang (Taiyang) or bladder, the Yangming (stomach) and Shaoyang (gallbladder) to the Taiyin (lungs), Shaoyin (kidneys) and Jueyin (liver), the patient will decline fairly rapidly. The symptomology mainly relates to the respective *zang* organs and their pathways. Treatment is first through sweating (up to the third day), and then, if more severe, through purging.

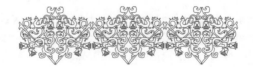

10. On Various Kinds of Pain

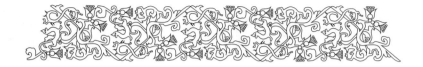

帝曰: 願聞人之五臟卒痛, 何氣使然?

岐伯對曰: 經脈流行不止, 環周不休, 寒氣入經而稽遲, 泣而不行.

客於脈外, 則血少, 客於脈中則氣不通, 故卒然而痛.

THE YELLOW EMPEROR ASKS, saying: I have heard that some people's bodies develop severe pain. What is it that brings this about?

Qi Bo replies, saying: The circulation in the channels and vessels moves on without stopping, encompassing the whole body without a break. When cold enters into a channel, it slows down this flow and delays it – the flow of the qi becomes uneven and they find it difficult to move. As cold lodges outside the vessel, the blood lessens; while when it lodges inside the vessel the qi cannot pass through freely, causing severe pain.

寒氣客於脈外, 則脈寒, 脈寒則縮踡, 縮踡則脈絀急,

則外引小絡, 故卒然而痛.

得炅則痛立止. 因重中於寒, 則痛久矣.

寒氣客於經脈之中, 與炅氣相薄, 則脈滿, 滿則痛而不可按也.

If cold lodges outside the vessel, the vessel grows cold; as it grows cold, it shrinks and contracts. Shrinking and contracting, the vessel is impeded and tightens; so then outside it involves the smaller subsidiary *luo* channels, causing severe pain. When warmed by the sun, the pain immediately stops. If the cold then attacks again, the pain is more lasting.

As the cold lodges in the channels and vessels, it grapples with the warm qi and the vessels feel blocked and full. Feeling blocked and full, they are so painful you cannot put your hand on them.

寒氣客於腸胃之間, 膜原之下, 血不得散, 小絡急引故痛.
按之則血氣散, 故按之痛止.
寒氣客於挾脊之脈則深, 按之不能及, 故按之無益也.

If the cold is lodged in the space between the outer surface of the skin and intestines, below the flat area of the fatty membranes, then the blood and qi cannot disperse and the small subsidiary channels tighten, leading to pain. You put your hand on them and the blood and qi disperse. So lay your hand on them, and the pain stops.

If the cold lodges in the vessels either side of the spine, even though you press deeply down with your hand you cannot reach it. Hence you press down on it, but there is no benefit.

寒氣客於衝脈, 衝脈起於關元, 隨腹直上, 寒氣客則脈不通.
脈不通則氣因之, 故喘氣應手矣.
寒氣客於背俞之脈, 則脈泣, 脈泣則血虛, 血虛則痛, 其俞注於心.
故相引而痛. 按之則熱氣至, 熱氣至則痛上矣.

If the cold is lodged in the Penetrating vessel, the Penetrating vessel arises from the 'source gate' and follows over the belly, travelling directly upwards. If the cold is lodged there, the vessel cannot flow freely. If the vessel cannot flow freely, nor does the qi follow its course, it causes difficulty in breathing – involving the arms.

If the cold is lodged in the vessel containing the back *shu* points, the vessel will become sluggish. If the vessel becomes sluggish, the blood weakens. As the blood is weakened there is pain, and the *shu* points move it into the centre of the body. This leads the pain on throughout. You lay your hand upon it and then the heat of your hand relieves it. As the heat relieves it, so the pain finally stops.

寒氣客於厥陰之脈, 厥陰之脈者, 絡陰器, 繫於肝.
寒氣客於脈中, 則血泣脈急, 故脅肋與少腹相引痛矣.
厥陰客於陰股, 寒氣上及少腹, 血泣在下相引, 故腹痛引陰股.

If cold is lodged in the Jueyin vessel, the Jueyin vessel is linked to the sex organs and ties up with the liver. If cold qi lodges in the vessel, the blood becomes sluggish and the vessel tightens – causing both ribs and lower belly to be in pain.

If weakening qi lodges in the inner thigh, cold rises to reach the lower belly, the blood becomes sluggish and leads on to pain throughout. Thus the belly pain leads down to the inner thigh.

寒氣客於小腸膜原之間, 絡血之中, 血泣不得注入大經,
血氣稽留不得行, 故宿昔而成積矣.

If the cold lodges between the small intestines and the flat area of the fatty membranes, in the subsidiary blood channels, then the blood flows unevenly and cannot circulate out into the larger channels. The blood and qi slow down, are held back and cannot circulate. Thus over a long period of time, they form accumulations.

寒氣客於五臟, 厥逆上泄, 陰氣竭, 陽氣未入, 故卒然痛.
死不知人, 氣復反則生矣.
寒氣客於腸胃, 厥逆上出, 故痛而嘔也.

If the cold lodges in the five *zang*, it causes weakening and the qi flows the wrong way, dissipating above. As the Yin qi brings exhaustion, the Yang cannot enter in, causing sudden pain. This creates a sudden collapse and you become unconscious. If the qi can be returned, you will certainly revive.

If the cold lodges in the intestines and stomach, it causes weakening – as the qi flows the wrong way above, causing pain and vomiting.

寒氣客於小腸, 小腸不得成聚, 故后泄復痛矣.
熱氣留於小腸, 腸中痛, 癉熱焦渴, 則堅乾不得出, 故痛而閉不通矣.

If cold lodges in the small intestines, they cannot complete their function of gathering in. This in time causes diarrhoea and then a painful belly.

If heat is retained in the small intestines, there is pain within the intestines. Then a numbed fever occurs, with a burning thirst, the stool becomes very hard, dry and cannot come out, causing pain and constipation as nothing is coming through.

This section is taken from *Suwen* 39, the same chapter which includes a discussion on the 'temperament' (see Section 7 earlier). It makes it clear that pain results from the blocked movement of the qi and blood in the channels, usually due to cold. Note, however, that the last three lines also indicate pain resulting from 'retained heat'. The text outlines several important factors: that when warmed by the sun the pain may stop, that putting your hand on the area may either aggravate or alleviate the pain (showing the depth of the problem). It describes cold coming to 'lodge' within the vessel, or outside the vessel, in the subsidiary *luo* channels, or between the skin and intestines, or below the fatty membranes (hyperchondium), or beside the spine, in the Penetrating vessel 冲脉 *chong mai*, in the back *shu* points, in the Liver Jueyin vessel, or in the inner thigh, around the small intestines, and so on. Symptomology is related to area and affected organ.

11. On *Bi* Immobility Syndromes

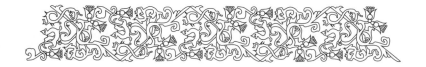

黃帝問曰: 痹之安生? 岐伯對曰: 風寒濕三氣雜至合而為痹也.
其風氣勝者為行痹, 寒氣勝者為痛痹, 濕氣勝者為著痹也.

THE YELLOW EMPEROR ASKS, saying: And now about *bi* immobility, how is that created? Qi Bo replies: The wind, the cold and the damp, these three climates arrive variously, but they all create *bi* immobility.

> Once wind qi predominates, you have travelling *bi*.
> Once cold qi predominates, you have painful *bi*.
> Once damp qi predominates, you have stubborn *bi*.

Li Zhongzi: *Bi* means closed off, it means numb. Among the six qi, wind, cold and damp are the malign Yin qi. The Yin qi together create the sickness, which implies that the imagery is of the obstructions which create the winter – the wind, cold and damp. Each causes the blood and qi to stop flowing, the Jingluo to get into stasis and close off. So this is how *bi* immobility syndromes are actually created.

肺痹者, 煩滿喘而嘔.
心痹者, 脈不通, 煩則心下鼓, 暴上氣而喘, 嗌乾善噫, 厥氣上則恐.
肝痹者, 夜臥則驚, 多飲, 數小便, 上為引如懷.
腎痹者, 善脹, 尻以代踵, 脊以代頭.
脾痹者, 四支解墮, 發咳嘔汁, 上為大塞.

When you have lung *bi*, it means anxiety and a feeling of fullness, breathlessness and, on top of this, vomiting.

When you have heart *bi*, it means the blood pulse is not coming through. There is anxiety, so a feeling of drumming under the heart. The qi violently ascends and you turn breathless. There is dry vomit and a tendency to belch. As the breath reverses above, so you are fearful.

When you have liver *bi*, it means at night you wake with a start. You drink often and frequently pass water. The rising qi leads to this, a feeling like something lodged in the belly.

When you have kidney *bi*, it means you are liable to become swollen. It seems to go from the tailbone down to the heels, from the spine down to the head.

When you have spleen *bi*, it means the four limbs feel tired and dropping. You produce a cough, bringing up fluid. The qi rises, causing a great obstruction.

腸痺者, 數飲而出不得, 中氣喘爭, 時發飧泄.

胞痺者, 少腹膀胱按之內痛, 若沃以湯, 澀於小便, 上為清涕.

When you have intestinal *bi*, it means you drink often but nothing passes out. Your *zhong* central qi causes difficulty in breathing and you struggle. At times, you pass undigested food in the stool.

When you have bladder *bi*, it means you lay your hand on the lower belly and bladder, and there is a pain felt within, as if scalded by hot water. There is a dragging sensation when you pass water, while above clear nasal mucus.

痛者, 寒氣多也, 有寒故痛也.

病久入深, 榮衛之行濇. 經絡時踈, 故不通. 皮膚不營, 故為不仁.

Pain means there is too much cold. There is cold, so it causes pain. If the sickness lasts a long time, the cold enters in so the circulation of the nutritive and defensive qi becomes uneven. As the Jingluo are dredged out, the pain goes. The skin and flesh are badly nourished, so it causes numbness.

陽氣少, 陰氣多, 與病相益, 故寒也.

陽氣多, 陰氣少, 病氣勝, 陽遭陰, 故為痺熱.

If the Yang qi is too little and the Yin qi too much, it reinforces the sickness, causing you to feel colder. If the Yang qi is too much and the Yin qi too little, the qi of the sickness is overpowered. The Yang confronts the Yin, causing *bi* and heat.

其多汗而濡者, 此其逢濕甚也. 陽氣少, 陰氣盛.

兩氣相盛, 故汗出而濡也.

凡痺之類, 逢寒則蟲, 逢熱則縱.

If there is so much sweat it drenches the body, it happens through encountering extreme damp. The Yang qi is too little and the Yin qi filled to excess. The two qi affect each other, making sweat and drenching you through.

With these differing types of *bi,* when you encounter cold there is a tightening; when you encounter heat, there is a slackening.

An interesting discussion of *bi* immobility 痺, caused through being affected by the wind, cold or damp, or even heat. Each of these malign factors can impede the free flow of the blood and qi. Wind leads to travelling *bi,* cold to painful *bi* and damp to stubborn *bi.* However, the obstruction may also involve the *zangfu* organs, including the lungs, heart, liver, kidneys and spleen, intestines or bladder. There is also a differentiation produced by Yin and Yang, cold, heat, sweating and the tone of the muscles.

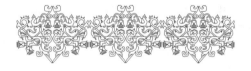

12. On Dreaming 1

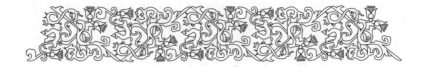

肺氣虛則使人夢見白物, 見人斬血借借. 得其時則夢見兵戰.
腎氣虛, 則使人夢見舟船溺人, 得其時則夢伏水中, 若有畏恐.
肝氣虛, 則夢見蘭香生草, 得其時則夢伏樹下不敢起.

WHEN THE QI OF THE LUNGS is weak,
It causes you to dream of seeing white things,
Of seeing men savagely cut down and bleeding.
At its moment, you dream of soldiers in battle.

When the qi of the kidneys is weak,
It causes you to dream of boats and drowning people.
At its moment, you dream of being submerged under water –
Perhaps of being scared and terrified.

When the qi of the liver is weak,
It causes you to dream of mushrooms and moulds,
And the fragrance of fresh grasses.
At its moment, you dream of being crouched under a tree,
Not daring to get up.

心氣虛, 則夢救火陽物, 得其時則夢燔灼.
脾氣虛則夢飲食不足, 得其時則夢築垣蓋屋.

When the qi of the heart is weak,
It causes you to dream of putting out a fire or drying things.
At its moment, you dream of a great blaze or conflagration.
When the qi of the spleen is weak,
It causes you to dream of eating and drinking
And not being satisfied.

At its moment, you dream of ramming down earth
For a wall or roofing over a dwelling.

WEAKNESS RESULTS IN DREAMING

weak organ	the dream
lungs	of seeing white things, men savagely cut down and bleeding, of soldiers in battle
kidneys	of boats and drowning people, of being submerged under water, perhaps of being scared and terrified
liver	of mushrooms and moulds, the fragrance of fresh grasses, crouched under a tree, not daring to get up
heart	of putting out a fire or drying things, of a great blaze or conflagration
spleen	of eating and drinking and not being satisfied, of ramming down earth for a wall or roofing over a dwelling

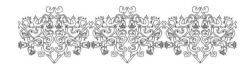

13. On Dreaming 2

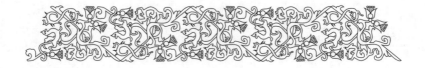

陰氣盛, 則夢涉大水而恐懼, 陽氣盛, 則夢大火而燔炳,
陰陽俱盛, 則夢相殺.
上盛則夢飛, 下盛則夢墮,
甚飢則夢取, 甚飽則夢予.

THE YIN QI FILLED, you dream of fording great rivers in
   trepidation.
The Yang qi filled, you dream of a great blaze and conflagration.
When Yin and Yang are both filled, you dream of mutual
   slaughter.
The body full above, you dream of flying.
The body weak below, you dream of falling.
If very hungry, you dream of getting.
If full of food, you dream of giving.

肝氣盛, 則夢怒, 肺氣盛, 則夢恐懼哭泣飛揚.
心氣盛, 則夢善笑恐畏, 脾氣盛, 則夢歌身體重不舉,
腎氣盛, 則夢腰脊兩解不屬.

The liver qi full, you dream of being angry.
The lung qi full, you dream of being fearful, of howling,
Of weeping tears, and a great disturbance!
The heart qi full, you dream of being happy and laughing,
Or of being frightened and scared.
The spleen qi full, you dream of singing joyfully,
The body feels heavy and you cannot get up.
The kidney qi full, you dream of waist and back
Being both loose and disconnected.

厥氣客於心, 則夢見丘山煙火.

客於肺, 則夢飛揚, 見金鐵之奇物.

客於肝, 則夢山林樹木.

客於脾, 則夢見丘陵大澤, 壞屋風雨.

客於腎, 則夢臨淵, 沒居水中,

客於膀胱, 則夢遊行, 客於胃, 則夢飲食.

客於大腸, 則夢田野, 客於小腸, 則夢聚邑沖衢,

客於膽, 則夢鬥訟自刳.

As the reversing qi is lodged in the heart,

So you dream of hills and mountains, and smoke from lit fires.

As it is lodged in the lungs,

So you dream of a great disturbance, and see strange objects of
  iron and gold.

As it is lodged in the liver,

So you dream of mountain forests, woods and great trees.

As it is lodged in the spleen,

So you dream of hills, mounds and the great marshes,

A hill-top house in the wind and rain.

As it is lodged in the kidneys,

So you dream of being at the brink of a steep cliff,

Of being lost or drowned in rivers.

As it is lodged in the bladder,

So you dream of travelling on or fording streams.

As it becomes lodged in the stomach,

So you dream of eating and drinking.

As it becomes lodged in the large intestines,

So you dream of barren and uncultivated fields.

As it becomes lodged in the small intestines,

So you dream of gathering on the busy highway.

As it becomes lodged in the gall,

So you dream of conflict and self-harming.

客於陰器, 則夢接內, 客於項, 則夢斬首,

客於脛, 則夢行走而不能前, 及居深地窌苑中.

客於股肱, 則夢禮節拜起, 客于胞䐈, 則夢溲便.

As it becomes lodged in the sex organs,
So you dream of sexual intercourse.
As it becomes lodged in the neck,
So you dream of the head being severed.
As it becomes lodged lower down,
So you dream of walking but not moving forward,
Or of being at a deep location or pit in the earth.
As it becomes lodged in the legs and arms,
So you dream of the restraints of ceremony and state.
As it becomes lodged in the lower belly,
So you dream of moving the bowels or passing water.

The two rightly famous sections above are on dreaming, one from the *Suwen* and the other from the *Lingshu*. Dreams, being akin to the imagination, are important for identifying underlying elemental conditions. Each of the five *zang*, when weak or being invaded, creates its own particular type of drama, and this idea extends also to a number of the *fu*. While the *Suwen* differentiates strictly by *zang* organs and speaks of weakness, the *Lingshu* gives the broader view. It speaks generally of fullness 'lodged' in the organ. These passages predate Freud's idea of 'wish-fulfilment' in *The Interpretation of Dreams* (1915) by some 2000 years. Note the phrase 'at its moment' 得其時 *de qi shi*, literally 'gain the time'. It is worth comparing this usage with the discussion of needling in Chapter VIII, Section 4. There it implies happenstance – that is, a mixture of circumstance and happiness which bring about a favourable outcome; in the section above it implies the moment of weakness within which creates the pathology of dreaming. See also the phrase 'its moment comes' in Section 15 below. All address the tangle of time involved as we reach between the pre-time and in-time worlds (see Appendix A). These chapters have also been much altered by later editors, but I have followed the NJZY and modern LSJJS edition for both.

FULLNESS RESULTS IN DREAMING

fullness in	the dream
the Yin qi	of fording great rivers in trepidation
the Yang qi	of a great blaze and conflagration
Yin and Yang	of mutual slaughter
full above	of flying
weak below	of falling
very hungry	of getting
full of food	of giving
liver qi	of being angry
lung qi	of being fearful, of howling, weeping tears and a great disturbance
heart qi	of being happy and laughing, or frightened and scared
spleen qi	of singing joyfully, the body heavy and you cannot get up
kidney qi	of waist and back being both loose and disconnected

THE REVERSING QI RESULTS IN DREAMING

lodged in	the dream
the heart	of hills and mountains, and smoke from lit fires
the lungs	of a great disturbance, and strange objects of iron and gold
the liver	of mountain forests, woods and great trees
the spleen	of hills, mounds and the great marshes, a hill-top house in the wind and rain
the kidneys	of being at the brink of a steep cliff, of being lost or drowned in rivers
the bladder	of travelling on or fording streams
the stomach	of eating and drinking
large intestines	of barren and uncultivated fields
small intestines	of gathering on the busy highway
the gallbladder	of conflict and self-harming
the sex organs	of sexual intercourse
the neck	of the head being severed
lower down	of walking but not moving forward, of being at a deep location or pit in the earth
legs and arms	of the restraints of ceremony and state
lower belly	of moving the bowels or passing water

14. Times of Dying: Channel Collapse

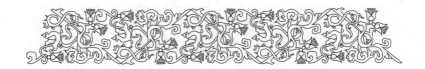

手太陰氣絕, 則皮毛焦. 太陰者, 行氣溫於皮毛者也.
故氣不榮, 則皮毛焦, 皮毛焦, 則津液去皮節,
津液去皮節者, 則爪枯毛折, 毛折者, 則毛先死.
丙篤丁死, 火勝金也.

WHEN THE HAND TAIYIN QI COLLAPSES, the skin and hair become dull and withered. The Taiyin circulates around the qi to warm the skin and hair. So this is how it is.

> As the qi is not able to nourish them,
> So the skin and hair become withered.
> The skin and hair withered,
> The fluids depart the skin and joints.
> As the fluids depart the skin and joints,
> Your nails wither and the hair on the skin breaks off.
> The hair on the skin breaking off means the body hair is first
>   to go.

At *bing* it worsens; and by *ting* it proves fatal. Fire overpowers metal.

The hand Taiyin is the Lung channel (metal), *bing* and *ting* indicate 'fire' days during the ten-day cycle.

手少陰氣絕, 則脈不通, 脈不通, 則血不流, 血不流, 則髮色不澤,
故其面黑如漆柴者, 血先死.
壬篤癸死, 水勝火也.

When the hand Shaoyin qi collapses, the blood vessels start not to
work well.

> The blood vessels not working well, the blood cannot flow.
> The blood unable to flow, the hair on the head loses its shine.
> So then your face becomes dark as lacquered black-wood
>   sticks.
> It is the blood which is first to go.

At *ren* it worsens; and by *gui* it proves fatal. Water overpowers fire.

The hand Shaoyin is the Heart channel (fire), *ren* and *gui* indicate 'water' days
during the ten-day cycle.

足太陰氣絕者, 則脈不榮肌肉. 唇舌者, 肌肉之本也.
脈不榮, 則肌肉軟, 肌肉軟, 則舌萎人中滿,
人中滿, 則唇反, 唇反者, 肉先死.
甲篤乙死, 木勝土也.

When the foot Taiyin qi collapses, the body vessels cannot nourish
the muscles and flesh. The lips and tongue are the root of the muscles
and flesh.

> The vessels not providing nourishment, the muscles and flesh
>   lose tone.
> The muscles and flesh losing tone, the tongue contracts
> And the upper lip is swollen above.
> The upper lip swollen above, the lips curl back.
> The lips curling back means it is the body flesh first to go.

At *jia* it worsens; and by *yi* it proves fatal. Wood overpowers earth.

The foot Taiyin is the Spleen channel (earth), *jia* and *yi* indicate 'wood' days
during the ten-day cycle.

足少陰氣絕, 則骨枯, 少陰者, 冬脈也, 伏行而濡骨髓者也,
故骨不濡, 則肉不能著也, 骨肉不相親, 則肉軟卻,
肉軟卻, 故齒長而垢, 發無澤, 發無澤者, 骨先死.
戊篤己死, 土勝水也.

When the foot Shaoyin qi collapses, so the bones wither. The Shaoyin is a winter vessel. It is hidden, circulating around, moistening the bone and marrow. This is what it does.

> So the bone not moistened, the flesh cannot manifest.
> If the flesh cannot manifest, the bones and flesh cannot relate
> And the flesh weakens and contracts.
> The flesh weakens and contracts means the teeth protrude
> And become stained, losing their shine.
> Losing their shine means it is the bones first to go.

At *wu* it worsens; and by *ji* it proves fatal. Earth overpowers water.

The foot Shaoyin is the Kidneys channel (water), *wu* and *ji* indicate 'earth' days during the ten-day cycle.

足厥陰氣絕, 則筋絕. 厥陰者, 肝脈也.
肝者, 筋之合也, 筋者, 聚於陰氣, 而脈絡於舌本也.
故脈弗榮, 則筋急, 筋急則引舌與卵, 故唇青舌卷卵縮, 則筋先死.
庚篤辛死, 金勝木也.

When the foot Jueyin qi collapses, the tendons also collapse. The Jueyin refers to the vessel of the liver. The liver is the union of the tendons. The tendons gather in the sex organs and their vessel links to the root of the tongue.

> So their vessel not nourished, the tendons go into spasm.
> The tendons in spasm contracts the tongue and scrotum.
> Then the lips turn greeny-blue, the tongue curls and the
>   scrotum shrinks.
> This means the tendons are the first to go.

At *geng* it worsens; and by *xin* it proves fatal. Metal overpowers wood.

The foot Jueyin is the Liver channel (wood), *geng* and *xin* indicate 'metal' days during the ten-day cycle.

五陰氣俱絕, 則目系轉, 轉則目運,
目運者, 為志先死, 志先死, 則遠一日半死矣.
六陽氣絕, 則陰與陽相離, 離則腠理發泄, 絕汗乃出.
故旦占夕死, 夕占旦死.

When all five Yin qi collapse together, it moves to the eyes.
Moving to the eyes means the look in the eyes changes.
The 'look in the eyes' changing means the will is first to go.
The will first to go, in a day and a half's time you perish.

When the six Yang qi collapse, Yin and Yang split apart.
As they split apart the pores of the skin break forth
In a heavy sweat which streams out.
This is the 'collapsing sweat' coming forth.
So: 'See it in the morning, by evening you are dead.
See it in the evening, by the dawn you are dead.'

The five Yin qi are of the *zang*, the six Yang qi are of the *fu*.

Finally, I have included some texts on 'times of dying'. These
are the last extracts in Li Zhongzi's *Cornerstone*, before the brief
section on 'the collapse of the channels' (see Section 16 below).
The above describes 'channel collapse' by linking symptoms to
the Lung hand Taiyin, Heart hand Shaoyin, Spleen foot Taiyin,
Kidney foot Shaoyin, Liver foot Jueyin, all five Yin and the six
Yang. The text clearly involves *wuxing* or *yinyang* reasoning. The
next section describes seasonal collapse and then, last, the collapse
of the channels. It describes the progression of disease at differing
times of the year: winter, spring, summer or autumn. In these
sections the notes between paragraphs – that act as an aid to
understanding the implicit reasoning in the text – are my own,
based on those of Li Zhongzi.

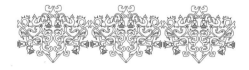

15. Times of Dying: Seasonal Collapse

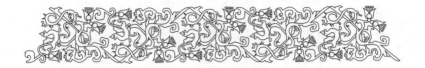

冬三月之病, 病合於陽者, 至春正月, 脈有死證, 皆歸出春.
冬三月之病, 在理已盡, 草與柳葉皆殺.
春陰陽皆絕, 期在孟春.

IN A SICKNESS SEEN during the three moons of winter, the sickness is 'enclosed in the Yang'. So then at the first moon of spring, the pulse starts to exhibit fatal symptoms. They both gather together at the opening of the spring.

In a sickness seen during the three moons of winter, there is no pattern to the symptoms. Then, as both the grass and willow green together, it means destruction.

During a spring when both Yin and Yang are faltering, its moment comes at the arrival of the first month of spring.

In spring, the Yang begins to rise; and the Yang sickness joins with it. Both Yangs 'gather together' and become overbearing. When both the 'grass and willow green together' it means full Yang. When 'both Yin and Yang are faltering', death does not even wait until the second month of spring.

春三月之病曰陽殺, 陰陽皆絕, 期在草乾.
夏三月之病, 至陰不過十日, 陰陽交, 期在溓水.

A sickness seen during the three moons of spring is called 'the Yang cut away'. With both Yin and Yang faltering, its moment comes at the withering of the grasses.

292

In a sickness seen during the three moons of summer, when it reaches the Yin, you will not last more than ten days. With both Yin and Yang undercut, its moment comes at the arrival of the torrential rains.

The 'withering of the grass' comes about as metal (autumn) overpowers wood (spring). Then its moment comes. The 'torrential rains' occur in autumn. In summer the Yin is in full retreat – if it becomes further invaded it cannot survive beyond autumn.

秋三月之病, 三陽俱起, 不治自己.
陰陽交合者, 立不能坐, 坐不能起. 三陰獨至, 期在石水.
二陰獨至, 期在盛水.

In a sickness seen during the three moons of autumn, the three Yang begin to be affected together. Even if not treated, it will be self-limiting and the patient will survive.

When Yin and Yang are both sick, you cannot sit down from standing, or get up from sitting. If three Yin arrive on their own, their moment comes when water freezes like a stone.

If two Yin arrive on their own, their moment comes at the first rains of spring.

In autumn the Yin is growing, so even with a sickness of the three Yang, Yang cannot overpower Yin. The disease is self-limiting. With Yin and Yang sick together, you just cannot move. With three Yin sick, a Yin sickness matches the Yin season. When two Yin are sick, the first rains and floods (Yin) bring aggravation and death.

The above sections on 'Times of Dying' give a sober reminder of the acute and sometimes poverty-stricken conditions under which much of Chinese medicine has flourished. As we read of the collapse of the channels, the suffering of the common people is very present. In this first section, *wuxing* reasoning is used by the physician to determine the hour or day of death. Here seasonal changes are identified as crucial to either recovery or succumbing to disease. Seasonal factors are too often neglected in modern practice. Again, my commentary below each paragraph follows that of Li Zhongzi.

16. The Collapse
of the Channels

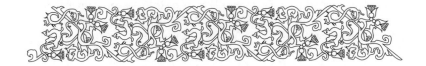

帝曰: 願聞十二經脈之終奈何? 岐伯曰:
太陽之脈, 其終也戴眼, 反折瘈瘲, 其色白, 絕汗乃出, 出則死矣.
少陽終者, 耳聾百節皆縱, 目寰絕系. 絕系一日半死,
其死也, 色先青, 白乃死矣.

THE YELLOW EMPEROR ASKS: What can you tell me about the
times when the twelve channels and vessels collapse?

Qi Bo replies: When it comes to the collapse of the Taiyang vessels,
the eyes flicker upwards, the back arches in convulsions, the
face turns white and the 'terminate sweat' comes out. When the
'terminate sweat' comes out, death is for certain.

When the Shaoyang vessels collapse, the ears go deaf; all the
joints slacken and let go; the eyes start out in terror and cannot move.
When the eyes cannot move, a day and a half and it proves fatal. On
death, the colour first becomes bluey-green. When the face turns
white, death is for certain.

陽明終者, 口目動作, 善驚妄言色黃. 其上下經盛, 不仁則終矣.
少陰終者, 面黑齒長而垢, 腹脹閉, 上下不通而終矣.

When the Yangming vessels collapse, the mouth and eyes tremble
and make small movements. They tend to start easily and the speech
becomes wild. The face turns yellow and the channels filled above
and below. When a numbness comes, it is at an end.

When the Shaoyin vessels collapse, the face turns black, the teeth
protrude and become stained. The belly swells up and is blocked up.
Nothing is moving through the body and death is for certain.

太陰終者, 腹脹閉, 不得息, 善噫善嘔, 嘔則逆, 逆則面赤,
不逆則上下不通, 不通則面黑, 皮毛焦而終矣.
厥陰終者, 中熱溢乾, 善溺心煩甚則舌卷, 卵上縮而終矣.

When the Taiyin vessels collapse, the belly swells up and is blocked
up. You cannot get a breath and tend to break wind and vomit, and
vomiting is the qi going against its usual course. As it goes against its
usual course, the face is flushed. Going against its usual course, above
and below, nothing is moving; as nothing is moving, the face turns
black. The skin and hair become dull and withered, and a collapse
is certain.

When the Jueyin vessels collapse, the centre of the body heats up.
Your throat gets dry and you tend to pass water. With an anxious
mind, you become restless. As it worsens your tongue stiffens, your
scrotum shrivels up and you finally collapse.

The collapse of the channels is introduced in order to bring home
again the drama of death. We progress systematically through
a discussion of the collapsing Taiyang, Shaoyang, Yangming,
Shaoyin, Taiyin and Jueyin vessels. Symptoms appear along the
course of the channel. Fatalities during treatment were common
before modern antibiotics; dying was an everyday affair. In
this whole chapter on pathology, 'associative' thinking and the
ubiquitous use of the *yinyang* or *wuxing* tool in the identification
and classification of disease is all-encompassing. Through
pondering these texts we can see directly into the workings of the
Chinese mind, struggling against the vagaries of a threatening
world. Xue Shengbai sums up the message, with his usual aplomb:

When a man is sick it is just as when a tree has grubs. Sickness
has its own pathology – just as grubs have a place they make
their own. If you do not know where they are hidden you may
hack at the whole tree and break it to pieces before they are

found and removed, and then the tree will die! If you do not know for certain where the sickness is, it spreads throughout the body, you treat it, the sickness feels no compulsion to depart, and life is finished! Therefore in pathology you must either reject or accept the evidence. But to do so may be as difficult as separating eye from eyebrow! You must do it in the fear of making the very slightest mistake. I cannot resist mentioning those who try a medicine when the pathology is not yet shown. These are the common hacks who boast of their families' traditional secrets. They are the followers of fashion who brag of a history containing any number of symptoms. They quarrel fiercely, disregarding the commonplace, not aware of their own limitations. Then they set forth their ideas of 'sickness from the three causes', with all possible variations, thinking any further discussion of the matter irrelevant! It is as if they did not even want to understand where the grubs were hidden – but would rather just hack at the tree and call it an achievement! Alas, how lamentable.

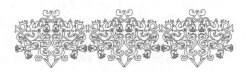

Questions for Review of Chapter IX
Indicates a more challenging question

1. Outline five or six commonly seen conditions, and explain how they relate to the *zangfu* or other elemental factors.

2. How might the seasons or diet affect the body's health?

3. Describe *in as much detail as possible* the five separate characters present in wood, fire, earth, metal and water people.

4. Explain how cold and heat work within the body according to *Suwen* 62.

5. What are the 'five full'? What are the 'five empty' or 'five weak'?

6. Describe *in a few words* how the qi moves in each of the following states: anger, happiness, sorrow, fear, cold, heat, being startled, tiredness, worry.

7. What is meant by the 'progression of fevers'?*

8. How are cold and pain related in the body?*

9. List as many kinds of *bi* syndrome as you can, with their main characteristics.

10. What kinds of dreams result from weakness in the five *zang*? What kinds of dreams accompany fullness? Expand on these ideas.

11. Explain how Yin and Yang are involved in the final collapse of the channels and death of the body. *

Characters in Chapter IX

strong or full 實 *shi*

weak or empty 虛 *xu*

six source qi: wind, cold, summer heat, damp, dryness and fire 六元氣 *liu yuan qi*

expelling 瀉 *xie*

tonifying 補 *bu*

eight principles 八綱 *ba gang*

cold injury 傷寒 *shanghan*

temperament 氣 *qi*

the Penetrating vessel 沖脈 *chong mai*

bi **immobility syndrome** 痺 *bi*

at its moment, gain the time 得其時 *de qi shi*

Appendix A

CLINICAL COSMOLOGY

The following six diagrams are given as an aid to working deeply with Yin and Yang. The evolution of the fluid Chinese ink brush during the Warring States and early Han – and the subscribing of signs and emblems to meaning – finally awoke the seeds of a *yinyang* philosophy. Yin and Yang represented the growth of ideas as well as passing of time. Black and white, day and night, light and shade, winter and summer, hot and cold, yes and no, right and wrong, full and empty, above and below – these allow us good clear sense (if we are up to it!) of the world as it is, and help us to become clear about 'physical dimension', 'the other', 'alteration and change' and 'our place in the world'.

A fluctuating self-reflective awareness of 'our place in the world' seems a good definition of the *yinyang*. This kind of meaningful ordering was no doubt brought about by watchers of the heavens and star-gazers. 'Heaven' was the source of blessing and good fortune. The falling rains promised a harvest to feed the people: heaven and earth (Yang and Yin), like benevolent parents, were joining in sending down blessings.

Through years working in a clinical setting I have sought for *greatness* as much as *health* in the person. The proper coming together of Yin and Yang in the body and its surroundings is often accelerated by moxa and the needle. After a few weeks of treatment, a patient's qi and blood are transformed – it can even happen in seconds.

The importance of acupuncture is that it actively boosts both identity and health. The instant of puncturing brings Yin and Yang to life! A biological imperative follows – a release of countless hormones and neurotransmitters flooding the body and brain. There is a sharpened awareness: the release of the 'original' or 'source' qi 元氣 *yuan qi* which seems, then, almost to 'stop time' – pointing towards a heightened consciousness, energy and well-being. This is to feel a boost to the body's immunity.

I find the best way to work with these occurrences (and one true to tradition) is to use the eight trigrams derived from *Yijing* science, which I mentioned earlier (see the Introduction). The genius of this clever system is that it allows the rapid interplay and run of Yin and Yang between sensation, symbolic lines and event, feeling and thinking. They are most decidedly *not conceptual* – yet also bound by logical rules. They allow the building of a clinical cosmology central to the Chinese tradition.

The first diagram below shows the *xiantian* or 'pre-time world' of the primitive. It depicts how Yin and Yang oppose each other as diametric opposites – 'heaven and earth in position, the mountain and marsh mixed together, thunder and wind stirring each other, water and fire passing each other through'. Second, in the *houtian* or 'in-time world', the trigrams are arranged to follow the march of the seasons. Time is the knot, as it were – which at once will bind the separate.

The third diagram expands on this view. The 'in-time' diagram depicts seasonal change – here it is explained further: spring ('thunder' and 'wind'), the heat of summer (as in 'fire', where the moist Yin is held within the Yang, ☲, as in a flower or berry), the fruits of late summer ('earth', mother, fullness), the destruction of autumn (the rotting lowlands or 'marsh') and severe winter (cold metal, dry skies, father); and then the deep, dark, cold days of the year ('water', with the dynamic Yang trapped within the Yin, ☵) and the stillness and quiet (of the settled 'mountain') before a rebirth in spring.

The fourth and fifth diagrams show a depiction of the waxing and waning moon; and then in my own 'brief style' I have sought to summarise each 'in-time' trigram in a single word. A certain daring, ubiquity and sense of the commonplace is intended. The broadest brushstroke may sometimes paint the best picture! I have found that 'sealing each trigram with a word' at a moment can be enormously therapeutic.

Use of the trigrams demands a study of the *Yijing* classics and perseverance. It is not obvious how Yin and Yang work. Yet I hope these dials from the old 'sky-lore' will help. They teach us how to restore and maintain the integrity of the Yang (health) – giving meaning, coherence and efficacy to our treatment. The last lines of the *Zhongyong* scripture, or *Doctrine of the Mean*, speak of needing balance in our work. Confucius, the master, quotes his favourite lines from the songs of the Zhou, describing the highest of human virtues:

> It is said in the *Book of Songs*: 'I regard with pleasure your bright virtue, making no great show of itself or colour. ' The Master commented: 'Show and colour are what transform the people – but this is nothing. ' The *Songs* also have a line: 'His virtue as light as a feather', although a feather still has some size. They also say: 'The workings of highest Heaven are without sound, or smell. ' Now this is best.

Perhaps if we attain to the finest needling, as a feather, along with the 'minutest of changes', we may aspire to such heights.

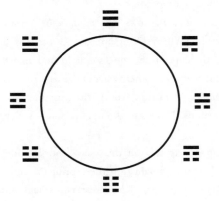

The *xiantian* or pre-time world

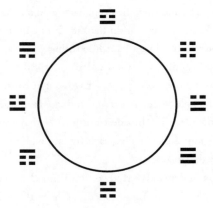

The *houtian* or in-time world

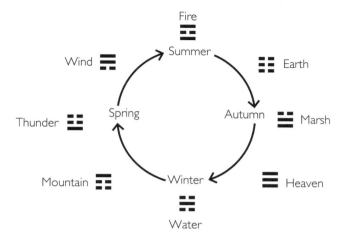

The 'in-time' trigrams and seasons

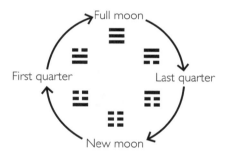

The moon of the in-time world

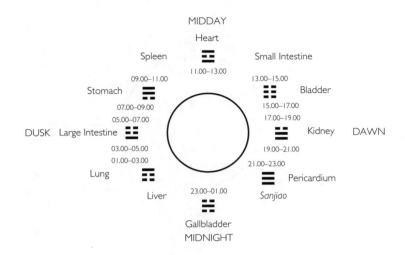

The daily clock and *zangfu* times

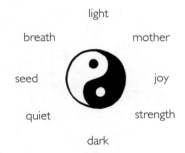

A 'brief style' for the in-time world

Appendix B

XUE SHENGBAI'S DISCOVERY
OF LI ZHONGZI'S WORK

I include below the original introduction by the renowned Xue Shengbai 薛
生 白 (1681–1770) to the reprinting of the *Neijing Zhiyao* (in 1764). Most
of the commentaries I include come from Li Zhongzi and Zhang Jiebin. The
brief afterwords for each chapter by Xue Shengbai have also been included. It
was Xue who saved Li Zhongzi's work from oblivion. The story is told in the
reprint about how he came down from his Buddhist retreat when he was 84,
and scoured the bookstalls in the local market, determined to find a copy of Li
Zhongzi's book. But the booksellers told him all had been lost and the wooden
printing blocks destroyed. So he had the original text recut anew, and reprinted.
This was the edition which survives to this day and is still used in China. His
hard-hitting introduction follows, with the characteristic implication that it is
only through fervent effort and study that we gain a deep and intuitive grasp of
the knowledge needed to practise:

> The Ancients used to say: for us humans to appreciate what it is to be
> human, we must understand medicine. These words would seem to indicate
> a particular clue to the meaning of friendship and filial piety. But what is it
> they really imply? As humans we are endowed with a physical body – but no
> explanation for it. The various evils, wind, fire, damp, summer heat, dryness
> and cold run through us without, while the emotions of joy, anger, worry,
> deliberation, grief and fright rampage around within – so, unless we know
> some restraint, it would be unusual if sickness did not make itself known.
> Well then, to be human must we put our parents, our uncles and brothers,
> wives and children, all of our household, into the hands of the Tang doctors,
> or should we not? If we should, then it is better we understand what it is
> they are saying.
>
> Now when understanding appears as understanding, all well and good.
> But when ignorance contrives to appear as understanding, this is not as
> good as understanding nothing at all! The whole business is ruined.

This generally describes that half-baked tradition which arises from the ignorance of those who are slaves to their own work. One such as this still has the stink of breast-milk about him! One day, by chance he gains command and through being at the right place at the right time, people load him with riches. Then he puts on a pompous and haughty air, employing medicine like a jailer with his prisoner, who acts contemptuously and makes as if medicine were hard work. When he hears that a household is sick, he hurries to treat them, taking the power of life and death into his own hands in order to impress. Has he never heard of Bianque, who said: 'I can revive them, but it is impossible to bring them back from the dead!' As to his medicine, he never thinks how, in the past, the Ancients divided medical practice into 14 disciplines and treated each as a speciality, their minds set upon aiding mankind.

Nowadays the rule for all is to copy from each other and follow fashion, running to the latest and best, and dabbling in it. Their minds are no more than watching out for recognition or calculating where the next meal is coming from, and this is all they do! Is this not the meanest behaviour?

It is crucial we understand the sources of our medical practice. They appear first in the discussion between the Yellow Emperor and his minister–physician where 'rightness in action' is taken as the single, sole aim. Indefatigably they have discussed the whys and wherefores of the people's sicknesses, handing down their teachings to all posterity that we might use suitable methods that accord with nature. And in addition herbal practice was first born with Emperor Shen Nong, who, through his own hard work and personal experience, examined the four seasons, and the suitability of soils and waters, hills and rivers. He tested the capabilities of all stones and minerals, and tasted the flavours of all plants, whether in streams or on dry land. Thereby he decided their functionality – which were toxic, which non-toxic, which were cooling, which heating, which warming, which bland or neutral, which attack, which reinforce, which slacken and which restrict.

This knowledge was passed on through the writings of the Yellow Emperor, and then entitled the *Suwen* (*Basic Questions*) and *Lingshu* (*Spiritual Crux*); and for Shen Nong it was contained in the *Bencao* (*Roots and Grasses*).

Since then any number of schools have appeared, besides Wang Bing's annotated commentary to the *Suwen*. As for the *Bencao*, in addition to

Tao Hongjing's *Mingyi Beilu* (*Miscellaneous Records of Celebrated Doctors*), successive generations of writers have come and gone. How is one to halt the sweating oxen who bear on their backs the cartloads of these books! They would fill a house to the rafters!

There is no remedy to these trend-setting teachers whose hearts are set on the byways of fashion. Vast numbers meet daily at court, or else decline an audience and withdraw, hoping then to be summoned and awarded the red silk girdle of office. Then they exchange presents in their local community, fearing that, if someone disapproves of their practice, they will be spoken ill of and lose business. Suddenly they come upon ceaseless calamities and then, day after day, cannot demean themselves enough, through cringing. Rest and food are dispensed with. How, then, will they have any time left for the tireless chanting and studying of the classics!

As a result of this, they carry about numerous satchels of books, books like the Li Shizhen and Zhang Jiebin compendiums. But there are none who do not gaze at these high cliffs and shirk back. How can they even come close to expressing the ideas behind that 'particular clue to friendship and filial duty'? Their hearts are filled with alarm. They feel a compulsion to go off at a tangent as soon as they understand. From an experience with one of their own family, they then indiscriminately love the whole world!

For a long time, I suffered the sloth of old age. Then, at last, in the year 1756, I withdrew into a monastery to live as a Buddhist monk. My lips are sealed and I do not talk about those days. Then one morning by chance, during my recollections, I remembered that the teacher Li Zhongzi had compiled several books. But it was only the *Neijing Zhiyao* (*The Cornerstone to the Neijing*) that came close to my own work – the *Yijing Yuanzhi* (*The Original Intention of the Medical Classics*) published in 1754.

It was Li Nianwo who allowed us to feel the Yellow Emperor and Qi Bo were our contemporaries – that is, to acquire the utter simplicity of knowledge and practice present in these two scrolls. Good work does not result from fashionable teachings. They are just the sound of a cock crowing at the lantern's light. You must rather have a standard and rule in your own breast. I asked at the book traders and they all said the printing blocks for Li Nianwo's works had long since been destroyed. But they urged me to have the blocks cut anew.

Alas, now! This book may fill a gap in your knowledge and its principles be gradually understood. It is exactly as if you carried a precious herb in your medicine basket, not knowing the old pathways or places it grew or where to pick it in season. Can medicine really be so easy to understand and practise? Yes, it can. But you must constantly make efforts not to court ignorance!

The year 1764 of Emperor Qianlong's reign. The 'Withered Old Herdsman' Xue Xue 薛雪 (Xue Shengbai) wrote this in his eighty-fourth year.

SELECT BIBLIOGRAPHY AND SOURCES

Primary Sources

Huang Fumi, *Zhejiu Jiayi Jing* (*ABC of Acupuncture and Moxibustion*). Beijing: People's Medical Publishing House, 1979. Originally published in 282 CE.

Lingshu Jing Jiaoshi (*A Checked Text with Explanations of the Lingshu Classic*). Hebei: People's Medical Publishing House, 1982. Mostly assembled c. 200 BC–200 CE. Abbreviated as LSJJS.

Li Zhongzi, *Neijing Zhiyao* (*A Cornerstone to the Neijing*). Beijing: People's Medical Publishing House, 1982. This is Li Zhongzi's original 1642 text with introduction and chapter notes by the Qing scholar Xue Shengbai, made in 1764. Abbreviated as NJZY.

Zhou Fengwu and Zhang Canjia, *Huangdi Neijing Suwen Yushi* (*The Huangdi Neijing in an Annotated Edition*). Shandong Scientific Publishing House, 1984. Mostly assembled c. 200 BCE–200 CE. Abbreviated as SWYS.

See http://ctext. org for the original *Huangdi Neijing* text.

Other Sources (in Chinese)

Gia-fu Feng (various dates, 1978–1980) Taped translation and transmission of the anonymous *Neijing Rumen* (*Introduction to the Neijing*). Hong Kong: Kwong Chi Book Company, no date.

Hsieh Kuan (Xie Guan), compiler and editor, *Chung-kuo I-hsueh Ta Tz'u-tien or Zhongguo yixue dacidian* (*Encyclopaedic Dictionary of Chinese Medicine*). Shanghai, 1921.

Ling Shu Jing (*Classic of the Miraculous Pivot*). Beijing: People's Medical Publishing House, 1979.

Neijing Rumen (*Introduction to the Neijing*). Hong Kong: Kwong Chi Book Company, no date.

Ou Ming, editor, *Han-Ying Chang Yong Zhongyi Cihui* (*A Chinese-English Glossary of Common Terms in TCM*). Guanggong: Science and Technology Press, 1982.

Qin Baiwei, *Neijing Zhiyao Qianjie* (*The Neijing Zhiyao Simply Explained*). Beijing: People's Medical Publishing House, 1985.

Tamba Motohiro (Tamba Genkan), *Suwen Shi, Suwen Shaoshi and Lingshu Shi*. Beijing: People's Medical Publishing Company, 1984. The Tamba commentaries made by the Japanese Tamba family, father Tamba Genkan, and sons Tamba Gen-in and Tamba Genken, in 1837, 1846 and 1808, respectively. From these, I have made the most use of the *Suwen Shi* (*Knowledge of the Suwen*). These most usefully quote the original Chinese commentators as well as being critical in their approach.

Zhang Jiepin, *Lei Jing* (*The Classified Classic*). Beijing: People's Medical Publishing House, 1964. Originally published in 1624. Zhang's approach was deeply influential on Li Zhongzi.

Zhongyi Renwu Cidian (*A Dictionary of Chinese Medical Personages*). Shanghai: Shanghai Literary Publishing House, 1988.

Other Sources (in English)

Allinson, Robert E. , *Understanding the Chinese Mind: The Philosophical Roots.* Oxford: Oxford University Press, 1989.

Beijing College of Traditional Chinese Medicine, *Essentials of Chinese Acupuncture.* Beijing: Beijing College of Traditional Chinese Medicine, 1980.

Bertschinger, R. , *Yijing: Shamanic Oracle of Change.* London: Singing Dragon, 2011.

Bertschinger, R. , *The Great Intent.* London: Singing Dragon, 2013.

Creel, H. G. with Chang, T. C. and Rudolph, R. C. , *Literary Chinese by the Inductive Method*, Vol. II. Chicago: Chicago University Press, 1979.

de Saussure, F. , *Course in General Linguistics*, trans. Roy Harris. Chicago, IL: Open Court Publishing, 1983.

Didier, J. C. , 'In and outside the square: The sky and the power of belief in Ancient China and the world, c. 4500 BC–AD 200. ' *Sino–Platonic Papers II*, p. 192 (September 2009).

Fung Yu-lan, *A History of Chinese Philosophy*, trans. Derk Bodde. Princeton: Princeton University Press. Vol. I: 1952, Vol. II: 1953.

Fung Yu-lan, *A History of Chinese Philosophy*. Princeton: Princeton University Press, 1983.

Hsu, E. , *The Transmission of Chinese Medicine.* Cambridge: Cambridge University Press, 1999.

Keegan, David Joseph, 'The *Huang Ti Nei Ching*: The structure of the compilation: The significance of the structure. ' PhD dissertation, University of Berkeley, 1988.

King, F. H. , *Farmers of Forty Centuries, or Permanent Agriculture in China, Korea, and Japan.* New York: Dover Publications, 2004.

Lan-yin Tseng, Lillian, *Picturing Heaven in Early China* (Harvard East Asian Monographs). Cambridge, MA: Harvard University Press, 2011.

Lee T'ao, 'Chinese medicine during the Ming dynasty (1368–1644). ' *Chinese Medical Journal 76*, 178–198, March 1958.

Levi-Strauss, Claude, *Totemism.* Boston: Beacon Press, 1963.

Levi-Strauss, Claude, *The Savage Mind.* Chicago: University of Chicago Press, 1966.

Levi-Strauss, Claude, *The Raw and the Cooked: Introduction to a Science of Mythology*, trans. John Weightman and Doreen Weightman. Vol. I of the *Mythologiques*. New York: Harper and Row, 1969.

Li Jingwei and Zhu Jianping, *An Illustrated Handbook of Chinese Qigong Forms from the Ancient Texts.* London: Singing Dragon, 2013.

Lin Yutang, *My Country and My People.* New York: Reynal and Hitchcock, 1935.

Ma Boying, *A Cultural History of Chinese Medicine.* In press; a translation of the *Zhongguo Yixue Wenhua Shi.*

Maoshing Ni, trans. , *The Yellow Emperor's Classic of Medicine: A New Translation of the Neijing Suwen with Commentary.* Boulder: Shambhala, 1995.

Merleau-Ponty, Maurice, *Phenomenology of Perception.* London: Routledge, 2013.

Needham, Joseph, *Science and Civilisation in China. Vol. II: History of Scientific Thought.* Cambridge: Cambridge University Press, 1956.

Plato, *Protagoras and Meno*, trans. Adam Beresford. London: Penguin Classics, 2005.

Smith, Brandley and Wan-go Weng, *China: A History in Art.* New York: Doubleday, 1979.

NOTES

Notes are listed by page and line number.

Introduction

15/16   **'correlative' thinking** There is a pointer to this type of thinking in Needham (1956), Vol. II, pp. 280–281.

15/21   **body's whole forces** Supreme 'ruler' or 'lord and master' 君主 *jun zhu* and 'military commander' 將軍 *jiangjun*, or general. Both examples are from Chapter V (below).

16/25   **David Keegan** mentions *Suwen* 4, *Suwen* 15, *Lingshu* 5 and *Lingshu* 28 as examples of this. See Keegan (1988).

17/3   **transmission under oath** Keegan (1988), p. 251.

17/9   *Neijing* Interestingly enough I was also told by my first acupuncture teacher Jack Worsley that my own classroom notes would form the best textbook I would ever have. Many of the appendices (or 'wings') to the *Yijing*, the ancient Zhou oracle, also seem to be classroom notes.

17/13   **create a lineage** This is not to deny, of course, that there was unity among them.

17/28   **post-revolutionary China (c. 1950s)** See Hsu (1999).

18/6   **Chinese thought** It was Han Feizi who supplied the legalist philosophy necessary for the later unification in 221 bce under the Emperor Qin Shi Huangdi.

19/28   **Qin (221–207 BCE)** This was 'the first emperor of all' or Shi Huangdi, who planned and built his own mausoleum filled with a lake of mercury and the famous 'Terracotta Army'.

20/8   **restorer of the old** 'I am a transmitter, not a creator, I love and cherish the ancients' (*Analects* VII: 1).

20/26   **'reciprocity' is the watchword** *Analects* XV: 24.

21/26   **serve their own parents** Both this and the foregoing quote are from *Mencius*, Book II, Part A, Chapter 6.

22/25   **Confucian canon** Added to this list should be also the canonical Daoist *Tao-te Ching* of Laozi and the *Zhuangzi*.

24/4   **Ma Boying** See Ma Boying (in press).

24/5   **'warring states' thinking** See Ma Boying (in press), Part II, Chapter 6. There is of course the well-known mention of the *wuxing* in the 'Flood Codes' ('Hong Fan') section of the *Book of History*.

24/7   **Zou Yan** His story is best told in Needham (1956), Vol. II, pp. 232ff.

24/20   **north and south** *Ibid.*

26/19   **month of the year** This selection is quoted in Fung (1983), Vol. 1, p. 164.

26/32   **flourishing and perishing of things** Beijing College of Traditional Chinese Medicine (1980), p. 11.

27/7   **treasury of a clear mind** See pages 81 and 192.

27/16   **'mutual interaction'** 相应 For more on 'mutual interaction' see Chapter I, Section 4, 'The Rhythm of the Seasons'.

28/3   **trigrams or hexagrams** This subject is followed up in detail in my translation *Yijing: Shamanic Oracle of Change* (Bertschinger 2011).

28/12   **they are lost** See page 151.

28/23   **One on its own sunken, is sickness** See page 124.

28/34   **Confucian and Taoist ideal** See page 60. Also at the end of the Confucian scripture *The Doctrine of the Mean* – a long passage eulogising the Sage.

29/8   **real people of substance** See pages 58–59.

29/23   **'equality of all things'** The term 'equality of all things' 齊物 *qiwu* comes from *Zhuangzi*, where it is the title of Chapter 2.

30/2   **remaining humble and empty** See page 56.

30/22   **just been reprinted** See Xue Shengbai's forthright preface, in Appendix B.

30/33   **'easy and simple'** The 'easy and simple', a byword for the operation of the *yinyang* within the *Yijing*.

31/21   **Kentang was cured** The story is from Hsieh Kuan (1921).

31/28   **Wu Youxing** See Lee T'ao (1958), p. 189.

32/16   **summary of important points** See Lee T'ao (1958), p. 179.

33/17   **early in the book** The phrase 'utter humility and a deep sense of peace' opens *Laozi* 16, and is clearly describing some kind of semi-meditative state: 'Obtaining utter humility, I guard a deep sense of peace: while all myriad things are created and I watch their rise and fall, they flourish, each one returning to its roots; as they return to their roots I am at peace. '

33/24   **the skies and the earth** Commentary to the *Neijing Zhiyao* (NJZY), Chapter I.

33/35   **life and death** Commentary to Chapter IV of NJZY.

35/4   **'cornerstone'** *Yao* 要 can mean 'key, cornerstone, crux, importance', and so on.

36/1   **the whole world** This distinction was first proposed by the great Neo-Confucian scholar Zhuxi (1130–1200).

36/12   **Buddha-nature, in all but name** Interestingly enough, this has more than a slight resemblance to Plato's thoughts on education in the Socratic dialogue with his disciple Meno. See Plato (2005).

36/20   **profundity of heaven** Fung (1983), p. 602. It may be an idea to substitute 'original goodness' for 'heaven'. The passage then reads somewhat more easily.

36/28   **Heavenly Principle (*tian li*)** This and the following quotes are from Fung (1983, Vol. 2), p. 606. Wang Yangming's interpretation called it 'the original state of our mind, which is spontaneously intelligent and keenly conscious' (quoted in Fung 1983, Vol. 2, p. 603).

37/21   **human devotion** Bertschinger (2011), page 59.

39/17   **image-language** Allinson (1989), p. 167.

40/4   **metaphysical contemplation** Allison (1989), p. 206.

40/16   **not a passive, task** Creel *et al.* (1979), p. 1.

41/22   **a trap for the meaning** This passage gets a slightly different translation in Fung (1983), Vol. 2, p. 184.

42/2   **facial diagnosis** See Chapter III.

42/4   **'rough, tough and hard' – not soft** See Chapter IV.

42/10   **patterns in treatment** See Chapter VII.

42/25   **that is, beyond words** In fact Levi-Strauss is representative of a continuous tradition leading back via Merleau-Ponty, Husserl and the rationalists Kant and Leibniz to China. The thought of Zhu Xi, as understood by the late Ming, was translated into Latin by the Jesuits and thus could be read in the 1670s by the young Leibniz, then in his early twenties.

42/29   *The Savage Mind The Savage Mind* should more accurately be translated as *The Untamed Mind*, with the implication that it is culture (that is, thought, language and so on) that makes all the difference.

43/14   **sensible intuition** Levi-Strauss (1966), p. 15.

43/26   *Mythologiques I, II, III, IV* Four giant volumes by Claude Levi-Strauss: *Mythologiques* (*The Raw and the Cooked*; *From Honey to Ashes*; *The Origin of Table Manners*; and *The Naked Man*). (First published in France, 1964–1971.)

44/13   **to finish a task** This of course has nothing to do with a 'botcher' – one who does a task in a bad or messy way. The words have different roots: 'bodge' is possibly cognate with 'fudge', and it works, while a 'botched' job does not. There is a small renaissance of bodgers in our Somerset neighbourhood.

44/18   **whatever he can find** See Levi-Strauss (1966), Chapter 1.

45/6   **black and white** A fact noted by Levi-Strauss (1963), p. 90.

45/7   **'binary oppositions'** The term is Ferdinand de Saussure's. See, for example, de Saussure (1983).

45/14   **'a logic of tangible qualities'** See Chapter 1 of Levi-Strauss (1969).

45/22   **form of propositions** Levi-Strauss (1969), p. 1.

46/3   **called the utensil** From the *Xici*, the canonical commentary on the *Yijing*.

46/9   **spirit in matter** And again this is illustrated in Appendix A through diagrams.

46/33   **Confucian** It also forms the backbone of the Taoist's physical, proto-biochemical yoga.

47/8   **'making the people anew'** This is how the Confucian *Great Learning* (*Da Xue*) expresses it. 'Making the people anew' is, of course, close to making them healthy and well.

47/23   **Kuang-ming Wu has said** Allinson (1989), p. 252.

48/10   **totally hidden** See Chapter IV, Section 4.

49/12   **in the West** See, for example, Hsu (1999).

50/7   **mysterious resonance** Needham (1956), Vol. V, p. 306.

50/16   **they know too much** *Laozi* 65.

Chapter I: The Arts and Ways of a Good Life

54/1   **The Yellow Emperor Questions his Counsellor** From 'The Natural Behaviour of Those of Ancient Times', *Suwen* 1.

55/20   **from Han times** The 'book' survives in two volumes, the *Suwen* (*Basic Questions*) and the *Lingshu* (*Spiritual Crux*). The latter was traditionally seen as heir to the oldest writings on acupuncture.

56/1   **A Message from the Ancients** From 'The Natural Behaviour of Those of Ancient Times', *Suwen* 1.

57/7   **I believe in and love the ancients** The Confucian *Analects* 1, 7.

57/25   **Confucian ethics** See also the opening to the Confucian primer *A Classic of Filial Piety* 孝經 or *Xiao Jing*, where we are told that even our 'body hair, and every bit of skin' should be constantly protected, as they were donated to us by our parents.

58/1   **They Represented the Arts and Ways of Life** From 'The Natural Behaviour of Those of Ancient Times', *Suwen* 1.

58/19   **When I no longer have a body, how can I suffer!** *Laozi* 13.

62/1   **The Rhythm of the Seasons** From 'On Regulating the Mind in Accordance with the Four Seasons', *Suwen* 2.

67/1   **The Energy of the Yang Stored up** *Ibid.*

70/1   **The Practice of Advancing the Yang** From 'On the Resonant Phenomena of Yin and Yang', *Suwen* 5.

70/13   **Li Dongyuan** Also known as Li Gao (1180–1252 ce).

71/1   **'nine openings'** Two eyes, two ears, two nostrils, a mouth and two lower openings.

71/32   **Zhuangzi** Chapter 18 title; and Chapter 21.

73/1   **Taoist Yoga** From 'Needling Methods', *Suwen* 72.

73/25   **Warring States** See, for example, Li and Zhu (2013).

74/2   **SWYS but is in the NJZY** SWYS and NJZY refer to two primary sources, the *Suwen Yushi* and *Neijing Zhiyao*. See Select Bibliography and Sources.

74/15   **firing an empty pan!** From his classical text *Wide Awake to Reality* (*Wuzhen Pian*).

75/1   **The Sages Treated those Well, not those Sick** From 'On Regulating the Mind in Accord with the Four Seasons', *Suwen* 2.

76/1   **The Character of the Malign *Xie* or Thief-Wind** From 'Nine Palaces, Eight Winds', *Lingshu* 77.

77/8   **an appreciation of 'place'** Didier (2009), pp. 20–21. This disc is also mentioned in Lan-yin Tseng (2011). Didier has produced a chart listing several early forms of the character *di* 帝, the classical symbol for 'ancient ruler' or 'king'. These early forms tend towards a four-fold or eight-fold symmetry, evoking a double dichotomy of direction and space, which could well be a depiction of the heavens. In other words, heaven above *is* our ruler. See diagram below.

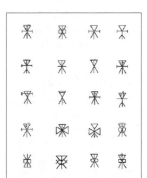

Early forms of the character *di* for ancient ruler
showing a clear four-fold or eight-fold symmetry

77/19   **watch what you eat** My own Chinese teacher, Gia-fu Feng, would have added more prosaically 'move your bowels'. The importance of catharsis and purging has always been fundamental to natural medicine.

79/8   **'easy and simple'** See note at 33/30.

Chapter II: Yin and Yang

81/1   **Yin and Yang, the Way of the Skies and Earth** From 'On the Resonant Phenomena of Yin and Yang', *Suwen* 5.

81/12   **Zhang Zhicong** A famous Qing dynasty commentator on the *Suwen*. Lived 1619–1674.

81/12   **the root in the Yin and Yang** This important concluding phrase is discussed further in Chapter VII, Section 1.

83/13   **the picture of change** The ideas of change are pursued in Appendix A.

83/32   **'investigation of things'** See page 37 in the Introduction.

84/6   **clear thinking** The more prosaic 'spiritual light' for *shenming* 神明 will not do. What emerges in this section is the criticality of the *yinyang* for clear thinking. Yin and Yang form a logical tool used to enable the mind to proceed. Li Zhongzi's commentary crystallises the antagonism which exists between spirit and world: on the one hand 'change and transformation unfathomable' 變化不測 *bianhua buce*, which is the province of the mind – and on the other hand 'materiality flowing into form' 品物流形 *pin wu liu xing*, the province of physical objects in the world. The one prefers movement, the other stillness; thus movement and stillness, Yin and Yang combine.

85/1   **Yin and Yang, Water, Fire, Qi and Flavours** From 'On the Resonant Phenomena of Yin and Yang', *Suwen* 5.

86/26   **oneness with nature** See the trigrams and diagrams in Appendix A. These are included for readers wishing to pursue the science of change and alchemical transformation further.

90/4   **fertility and development** The term *jing* 精 can also have the meaning of 'sperm' or 'seed'.

92/1   **Left and Right as different as North and South** From 'On the Resonant Phenomena of Yin and Yang', *Suwen* 5.

94/1   **Yin and Yang in the Skies and Man** From 'The True Texts Stored within his Golden Casket', *Suwen* 4.

97/1   **The Crucial Importance of the Yang Needing Rest** From 'On Life Energies which Permeate the Natural World', *Suwen* 3.

98/9   **a truth in all nature** The *Wenyan* commentary on the *Yijing* says, 'The Sage arises and all creatures follow him with their eyes. '

98/28   **contained and protected** The work of the *ying* (nutrient; more Yin) and *wei* (defensive; more Yang) qi shows also the activity of the *yinyang*.

Chapter III: Examining the Colour

102/1   **Purity, Brightness, Colour and Complexion** From 'The Importance of the Pulse and its Deteriorating Purity', *Suwen* 17.

102/6   **Wu Kun** Famous Ming commentator on the *Suwen* (lived 1552–1620).

102/11   **scarlet silken wrapping** Following the NJZY in reading 帛 'silk' here, not 白 'white, plain'.

102/22   **a deteriorating purity in the five colours is** Following the interpretation by Yu Lun (1862–1919) here, as recommended by the modern SWYS editors.

105/1   **The Bright-lit Hall, the Physiognomy of Face** From 'The Five Colours', *Lingshu* 49.

111/22   **'monarch of the face'** The 'monarch of the face' is the tip of the nose. See page 108.

114/1   **The Basis of Health in the Face** From 'Five *Zang* from Birth to Completion', *Suwen* 10.

115/3   **is well testified** See the much reprinted *Farmers of Forty Centuries, or Permanent Agriculture in China, Korea, and Japan* by the American agronomist F. H. King (2004).

Chapter IV: The Quiet Pulse

120/1   **The Method of the Pulse Exam** From 'The Importance of the Pulse and its Deteriorating Purity', *Suwen* 17.

120/7   **Yang qi not yet scattered** Following the NJZY; the SWYS editors interchange Yin and Yang in this sentence.

120/21   **Ma Shi** Late Ming commentator on the *Suwen*.

121/22   **Hua Shou** Late Yuan/early Song physician. Wrote *Elucidations of the Fourteen Jing* (1341) with excellent diagrams; also the *Du Suwen Chao* (*Copied-out Passages from the Suwen*) – see the Introduction.

124/1   **If a Single Pulse Stands Out** From 'The Three Regions and Nine Climes', *Suwen* 20.

125/1   **The Primacy of the Pulse** From 'Aspects of Thriving and Declining Energies', *Suwen* 80.

126/1   **In Attending to the Pulse** From 'The Importance of the Pulse and its Deteriorating Purity', *Suwen* 17.

126/15   **the *junzi*** The Confucian ideal, or 'gentleman' scholar.

128/1   **In Spring, the Pulse is in the Liver** From 'The Uniquely Precious Workings of the True *Zang*', *Suwen* 19.

133/1   **The Healthy, Sick and Fatal Pulses** From 'The Character of the Qi in Healthy People', *Suwen* 18.

138/1   **The Arrival of the Fatal Pulse** From 'On Extreme Oddities', *Suwen* 48.

139/6   **jujube** The jujube tree or Chinese date.

141/32   ***ping*-fire declines at *wu*-earth** On *ping* (fire) and *wu* (earth) see Chapter IX, 'Pathology'.

143/1   **The Ultimate Tool** From 'Guiding the *Jing*, Reforming the Qi', *Suwen* 13.

144/5   **common in classical texts** See the opening paragraph to the Confucian *Da Xue* (*Great Learning*), and also Heshang Gong's early commentary to the *Tao-te Ching* (or *Laozi*), where the body is seen as a caricature of the state.

145/1   **A Common Fault in the Pulse Exam** From 'Clear Evidence of Four Failings', *Suwen* 78.

146/8   **Xu Shuwei** Lived 1079–1154.

Chapter V: The Zangfu and Wuxing

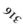

150/1   **The Offices of the** Zangfu From 'The Secret Codex from His Most Magic Writings', *Suwen* 8.

150/14 **'middle of the chest'** The 'middle of the chest' 膻中 *shanzhong* here refers to the area surrounding the heart. See page 154.

151/5   ***sanjiao*** The 三焦 *sanjiao* is the term for the 'three heating-spaces' of the body.

152/1   **future generations** '*Ling*' 靈 can mean 'spiritual', as well as 'most magical' and 'marvellous'. It is the same character as that in the title of the second volume of the *Neijing*: the *Lingshu*.

153/1   **The Zang and their Associations** From 'The Six Seasonal Divisions and Imagery of the *Zang*', *Suwen* 9.

153/10 **the Taiyang** On Taiyin, Taiyang and so on, see Chapter VI, 'Channels and Collaterals'. Some editors disagree about the Taiyang, Taiyin, Shaoyang and Shaoyin namings in this section.

154/1   ***hun* soul** 魄 *po* soul and 魂 *hun* soul are the Yang and Yin souls respectively.

154/17 **'four whites' by the lips** 'Four whites' 四白 *sibai*, now known as acupoint St 2; but Li Zhongzi says 'four whites' refers to 'the boundary of paler flesh surrounding the lips'.

156/1   **Directions and Elemental Associations** From 'The True Texts Stored in his Golden Casket', *Suwen* 4.

157/6   **'zhi'** Some sources sound this note '*zheng*'.

158/22 **'mysterious mutual mixing'** This is an attempt to translate 神秘互渗 *shenmi hushen*. According to new researches by Professor Ma Boying, a mysterious or mystical mutual permeation underpinned the growth of early Chinese medicine, especially the *Suwen*. The term might be best rendered 'strange interaction'. See Ma Boying (in press).

158/25 **eco-logic** The 'body ecologic' is an idea developed by Professor Elisabeth Hsu.

159/1   **Further Elemental Forms and *Wuxing* Science** From 'On the Resonant Phenomena of Yin and Yang', *Suwen* 5.

159/16 **the 'five tastes'** The sour, bitter, sweet, pungent and salty flavours.

163/4   **commonplace in early medicine** Again, see Ma Boying (in press).

164/16 **'grasp. . . it cannot be held'** *Laozi* 14.

164/17 **feelings bind us to the concrete** It is interesting that the French existentialist Merleau-Ponty reached quite a similar viewpoint in his *Phenomenology of Perception* (Routledge London 2013). The Chinese character *li* (see page 35 in the Introduction) also suggests a 'felt perception' or physical merging with 'unlettered' experience. This parallels the Gestalt idea of 'excitation' or direct contact of the human organism with his/her environment. This was a point not lost on my Chinese teacher Gia-fu Feng, who himself worked with Fritz Perls, the founder of Gestalt therapy, during the 1970s. It also echoes the Taoist ideal of 'energy and ecstasy' (for instance, in the book *Zhuangzi*) – the expanding of the individual self until lost in the world. I am reminded of the Zen story of the monk who lay dying: just as he goes, a bird sings out, close to him – 'Just that!' he says. 'Just that!'

165/3   **Pentatonic Tone, Element and Aspect** Based on 'The True Texts Stored in his Golden Casket', *Suwen* 4.

166/1   **Five Directions with Traditional Associations** Based on 'The True Texts Stored in his Golden Casket', *Suwen* 4.

167/1   **The Faculties of the Self, and their Injuries** From 'The Fundamentals of the Spirit', *Lingshu* 8.

170/1   **Physical Functions in Life and Death** From 'Determining Differing Kinds of Qi', *Lingshu* 30.

172/32   **and await the hare!** The implication is that meaning will get caught in words, just as a hare is caught in the trap. Compare Wang Bi's image involving the 'fish trap' on page 41.

Chapter VI: Channels and Collaterals

176/1   **The Form and Length of the Channels** From the chapter 'On the Channels and Vessels', *Lingshu* 10. In this chapter the titles of the channels may be translated as Taiyin 'Greater Yin', Taiyang 'Greater Yang', Yangming 'Brightest Yang', Shaoyang 'Lesser Yang', Shaoyin 'Lesser Yin' and Jueyin 'Absolute Yin'.

176/17   **'inch-wide mouth'** The area of the radial pulse.

176/19   **'fish'** Lu 10 *Yuji*, over the thenar eminence.

177/9   **'joining valleys'** LI 4 *Hegu*.

177/17   **'column bone'** The seventh cervical spinal process.

177/20   **'broken basin'** St 12 *Quepen*.

177/24   **'middle man'** Du 26 *Renzhong*.

178/7   **'receiving fluid'** Ren 24 *Chengjiang*.

178/9   **'great welcome'** St 5 *Daying*.

178/10   **'cheek carriage'** St 6 *Jiache*.

178/11   **'guest and host'** GB 3 *Kezhu*.

178/15   **'people welcome'** St 9 *Renying*.

178/21   **'qi highway'** St 30 *Qijie*.

178/25   **'thigh pass'** St 31 *Biguan*.

178/26   **'crouched rabbit'** St 32 *Futu*.

179/9   **'walnut bone'** The head of the first metatarsal.

180/4   **'joy bone'** The pisiform bone in the wrist by the acupoint He 7 *Shenmen*.

181/33   **'capital bone'** Bl 64 *Jinggu*.

182/9   **'blazing valley'** K 2 *Rangu*.

184/25   **'jawbone joint'** St 6 *Jiache*.

185/2   **'supporting bone'** The tibial crest.

185/3   **'terminate bone'** *Juegu*, another name for GB 39 *Xuanzhong*.

186/10   **'central pole'** Ren 2 *Zhongji*.

186/12   **'pass primal'** Ren 4 *Guanyuan*.

186/27   **'crossing space'** Possibly the area above the perineum, Ren 1 *Huiyin*.

186/29   **Huge Yang** Refers to the Bladder foot Taiyang.

187/8   **the 'crossing'** The same as 'crossing space', above.

188/9   **twenty-seven qi** The 12 channels 經 *jing*; the 12 collaterals 絡 *luo*; the *Du* Governor and *Ren* Conception vessels; plus the single great collateral of the Spleen hand Taiyin.

Chapter VII: Patterns of Treatment

192/1 **Yin and Yang, the Rule and Pattern** From 'The Resonant Phenomena of Yin and Yang', *Suwen* 5.

192/21 *Huainan Zi* An early Taoist scripture by Liu An, dated to around 140 BCE.

193/7 **Yin and Yang remain the root** See the opening section of Chapter II, 'Yin and Yang'.

193/12 **in the Introduction** See pages 36–37.

194/1 **The Seed in Sickness** From 'The Grand Discourse of Ultimate Truth and Importance', *Suwen* 74. Li Zhongzi runs this passage straight on from my former selection, without acknowledging that it comes from a separate chapter. Possibly his text conflated the chapters.

195/31 **hot medicines to treat a cold sickness** See Section 5, 'Treatment with Herbals, Foodstuffs and Flavours'.

196/1 **Mind, Body and Disease** From 'Blood, Qi, Body and Mind', *Suwen* 24.

196/17 **in the throat and insides** Huang Fumi's *ABC of Acupuncture and Moxibustion* here writes 'from absolute exhaustion'. I follow the SWYS reading.

198/1 **Regional Types, Regional Medicines** From 'How Treatments Differ According to Region', *Suwen* 12.

198/8 **heaven and earth first come into being** Possibly because it is where the sun rises.

199/10 **'poison herbs'** 'Poison herbs' 毒藥 *duyao* or, perhaps better, 'drastic herbs' is the old name for herbal medicines.

200/1 *bi* **immobility** *Bi* 痺 means 'obstruction, immobility'. The symptoms are pain, numbness and so on. See Chapter IX, Section 9, 'On *Bi* Immobility Syndromes'.

202/1 **Treatment with Herbals, Foodstuffs and Flavours** From 'The Grand Discourse of Ultimate Truth and Importance', *Suwen* 74.

204/32 **Ma Shi** Late Ming physician. Produced his *Huangdi Neijing* Zhuzheng Fawei in 1586.

205/22 **both may be sought in the kidneys** 'Single water', a 'single fire', also commonly called Kidney Yin and Kidney Yang respectively.

205/23 **Wang, our Great Teacher** Wang Bing.

208/1 **How Foodstuffs and Medicines can do Harm** From 'The Grand Discourse of Ultimate Truth and Importance', *Suwen* 74.

209/1 **Therapeutic Actions, How to Treat** From 'On the Resonant Phenomena of Yin and Yang', *Suwen* 5.

211/1 **'according to kind'** See pages 195 and 205–206.

211/3 **'overcome the main part'** See pages 204–206.

212/1 **Five Faults Made during Treatment** From 'Elucidating the Five Faults', *Suwen* 77.

215/1 **The Ultimate Task** From 'Guiding the *Jing*, Reforming the Qi', *Suwen* 13.

216/19 **'the five within'** The five *zang* organs.

216/20 **'bright-lit hall'** The central part of the forehead. See Chapter III, 'Examining the Colour'. Here Xue Shengbai lists the achievements of Li Zhongzi's previous five chapters, on Yin and Yang, colour and pulse, the *zangfu* and Jingluo.

Chapter VIII: *The Method of Needling*

221/1   **Origins of Five Element Acupuncture** From 'The Precious Life Force in the Whole Body', *Suwen* 25.

222/9   **the simple people of the Jin** The Jin existed 897–221 BCE, after which they grew to overthrow all other states and establish the Jin dynasty. Qi Bo is referring to the simple, hard-working village people to whom it never occurred to learn the art of the needle.

222/29   **what all practitioners totally understand** This passage really shows how simple acupuncture can be. It is the timing and graduation of effort which is critical. My own teacher summed it up: 'The single most pressing problem is learning how hard to push. ' To feel the beat of the universe, inside and out, and work to either resonate or disunite – all have their aim in creating harmony. Zhang Jiebin here refers to the attitude of the Taoist storyteller and philosopher Zhuangzi.

223/24   **flesh and outsides hold together** There is quite some difficulty in reading this passage. I read 肉 for 內, as suggested by the excellent resource of the Chinese Text website http://ctext. org.

224/23   **emphasise weakness** Which is to say, 'Needling weakness, watch for the filling of the qi. Needling fullness, watch for the emptying and clearing of the pathogen. '

224/24   **do not lose it** By extension this could also imply 'Guard the moment! Do not lose it!'

225/31   **you 'cannot properly fathom it'** A part of this evocative passage was included in my earlier book *The Great Intent* (Bertschinger 2013).

226/1   **Opening Chapter of the *Lingshu*** From 'The Nine Needles and Twelve Sources', *Lingshu* 1.

227/26   **the spirit, yes we must understand the spirit!** I translate this famous phrase '*shen hushen*' slightly differently in Chapter VII, Section 7, as 'the spirit is the spirit!'

229/14   **to go against** Reading 逆 instead of 迎, as suggested in the LSJJS.

231/1   **The Method** From 'The Eight Proper Sections and a Clear Mind', *Suwen* 26.

232/14   **east, south, west, north, southeast, southwest, northeast and northwest** Compare the description of the winds in Chapter I, Section 9, 'The Character of the Malign *Xie* or Thief-Wind', and diagrams in Appendix A. Inappropriate weather is seen to engender imbalance, and thus disease.

233/1   **Acupuncture: Treatment by Sun, Moon and Planets** From 'The Eight Proper Sections and a Clear Mind', *Suwen* 26.

236/1   **He Who Observes the Minutest of Changes** *Ibid.*

237/20   **參 伍 *canwu* has been discussed earlier** See Chapter IV, Section 1, 'The Method of the Pulse Exam'.

238/1   **Acupuncture: Technique, Reducing and Reinforcing** From 'The Eight Proper Sections and a Clear Mind', *Suwen* 26.

239/32   ***Lingshu* passages below** From 'On Capabilities', *Lingshu* 73.

241/1   **Acupuncture: What is Meant by the Spirit** From 'The Eight Proper Sections and a Clear Mind', *Suwen* 26.

243/1   **Four Common Failings in Treatment** From 'Clear Evidence of Four Failings', *Suwen* 78.

Chapter IX: Pathology

248/1   **A Typology of Conditions** From 'On the Essentials of Utter Truth', *Suwen* 74.

251/1   **Elemental, Seasonal and Dietary Injuries** From 'On Life Energies Which Permeate the Natural World', *Suwen* 3.

254/1   **Elemental Forms and Body Isomorphism** From 'On Yin and Yang in the Twenty-five Types of People', *Lingshu* 64.

254/14   **foot Jueyin** The Liver foot Jueyin.

255/10   **hand Shaoyin** The Heart hand Shaoyin.

255/26   **foot Taiyin** The Spleen foot Taiyin.

256/9   **hand Taiyin** The Lung hand Taiyin.

256/25   **foot Shaoyin** The Kidney foot Shaoyin.

257/2   **the *Lingshu*, probably the earliest** My definitive text is the contemporary Hebei medical college edition, the LSJJS.

259/1   **A Complete Explanation of the Full or Weak** From 'A Total Understanding of Weak and Strong', *Suwen* 28.

262/1   **Cold and Heat, Yin and Yang, Inner and Outer** From 'A Discourse on Regulating the Channels', *Suwen* 62.

265/1   **The Five Full, the Five Weak** From 'The Mechanism of Utmost Preciousness in the True Organs', *Suwen* 19.

267/1   **On the Temperament** From 'A Discourse on Attending to Pain', *Suwen* 39.

270/1   **How Heat Represents in the Face** From 'Needling Hot Conditions', *Suwen* 32.

272/1   **On the Progression of Fevers** From 'A Discourse on Fever', *Suwen* 31.

275/1   **On Various Kinds of Pain** From 'A Discourse on Various Painful Conditions', *Suwen* 39.

279/1   **On Bi Immobility Syndromes** From 'A Discourse on Bi', *Suwen* 43.

282/1   **On Dreaming 1** From 'The Plan in Filling and Declining', *Suwen* 80.

284/1   **On Dreaming 2** From 'On the Wild and Malign developing as Dreams', *Lingshu* 43.

288/1   **Times of Dying: Channel Collapse** From 'The Jingmai', *Lingshu* 10.

292/1   **Times of Dying: Seasonal Collapse** From 'A Discourse on the Principles of Yin and Yang', *Suwen* 79.

294/1   **The Collapse of the Channels** From 'A Critical Examination of the Jing Collapse', *Suwen* 16.

Appendix A: Clinical Cosmology

298/29   **the body's immunity** As a classical example of this see the poem in my earlier book, *The Great Intent* (Bertschinger 2013).

299/2   **logical rules** See the quotation from Wang Bi in the Introduction.

299/7   **passing each other through** A quotation from the *Shuogua*.

299/37   **now this is best** Quotation from *Zhongyong*, Chapter XXXIII, Section 6.

Appendix B: Xue Shengbai's Discovery of Li Zhongzi's Work

304/9   **Bianque** A legendary figure.

304/20   **the single, sole aim** In other words, in the *Huangdi Neijing*.

304/24   **Shen Nong** The legendary herbalist.

305/2   **generations of writers have come and gone** Tao Hongjing lived 456–536 CE.

306/7   **in his eighty-fourth year Xue** Xue, also known as Xue Shengbai, physician and writer of the Qing, lived AD 1681–1770, reaching the great age of 89.